Food Maintenance

by Carmella Irick

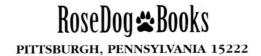

PITTSBURGH, PENNSYLVANIA 15222

The contents of this work including, but not limited to, the accuracy of events, people, and places depicted; opinions expressed; permission to use previously published materials included; and any advice given or actions advocated are solely the responsibility of the author, who assumes all liability for said work and indemnifies the publisher against any claims stemming from publication of the work.

All Rights Reserved
Copyright © 2009 by Carmella Irick
No part of this book may be reproduced or transmitted in any form or by any means, electronic or mechanical, including photocopying, recording, or by any information storage and retrieval system without permission in writing from the author.

ISBN: 978-1-4349-9358-8
Printed in the United States of America

First Printing

For more information or to order additional books,
please contact:
RoseDog Books
701 Smithfield Street
Pittsburgh, Pennsylvania 15222
U.S.A.
1-800-834-1803
www.rosedogbookstore.com

Chapter One
Self-Reflection

Food Maintenance is holistic approach to better eating and living habits; by understanding the root cause of the Compulsive Overeating behaviors that have develop over time; and recognizing the need for internal lifestyle changes. Learning how to eat and understanding that your emotional state is a major factor involved in the overeating process; the philosophy of Food Maintenance is holistic by design, in order for you to make the body, mind and spirit connection, and view all life areas as one entity, they are intertwined; and what affects one, affects the other.

The FM philosophy is based on five unifying concepts; this include;

1. Self-Actualization: Good health and maintaining health begins and ends with you making a commitment to your self mind, body, and spirit.
2. Developing and enhancing a positive and proactive attitude "Yes I can and I will"
3. The realization that You have the power and ability to discontinue this negative unhealthy relationship with food, by not allowing your negative self to dictate how you eat and/or abuse food during crisis, and emotional pitfalls i.e. relationship, fiancés, loneness, melancholy, depression,
4. Making the mind, body and spiritual connection to assist /facilitate a sense of well-being during good and difficult periods
5. Understanding/Accepting that what you put in you must be willing to work for.

The purpose of food Maintenance is to assist you with confronting yourself regarding how you use food and to promote discipline regarding your specific eating pattern. What I have learned over the years is that, healthy eating is only half of the equation. For ideal health, your body needs to be physically active with a focus; specifically on toning muscles, and burning calories. Slowly reduce your portion sizes, and start slowly and gradually to increasing your activity. And this doesn't necessarily mean hard exercise, walking, housework; gardening and running around with your kids can lead to healthy changes in your fitness level.

In order for positive changes to occur you must begin to work on your inner self, and build your self-esteem. In addition to focus on how you see yourself and where you see yourself.

Change is internal not external; and for most people, eating is a pleasurable experience. It's a biological necessity; However, Compulsive Overeaters use food inappropriately and eventually become addicted to it, and lose control over the amount of food they eat; due to anticipation of pleasure from the ingestion of food.

Overeaters present with moderate to severe obesity; and obesity causes childhood obesity increased childhood diabetes, heart conditions; there has been a significant increase with women having heart attacks due to increased Cholesterol. DIET; simply don't work because they force you to deprive yourself; there is so much confusing information out there today; therefore, it's very understandable when people become discouraged about selecting an eating plan for themselves. Most over eat because their unhappy, or unsatisfied with self and/or present /past life situations.

Conditioning: Simply means learned behaviors, i.e. your family of origin; reflect on your family, your culture, economic status, and race; yes this plays a major role in how and what each individual eats. For some families faith and food go hand in hand, and for some the use of food was/is interchangeable; celebrations weddings graduations, good grades, and used as a gift for lack of money i.e. bake a cake cookies ect; during negative periods i.e. Funeral, divorce, separations, a cheating partner, spouse, a child in trouble, eating to avoid negative feelings, and emotions, ect,.

The Emotional Pit Falls/Situations: Most over eat /abuse food due to stress, depression, melancholy, and relationships concerns; these are major factor in the over eating process; we all want and need to be loved, and too feel appreciated, and when that is missing something must fill that void in these sensitive life area; and **Food** has a tendency to be that constant; the one thing that you feel won't fail you. "Stop looking for outside validation, you have value, and purpose". At some point you have allowed your feelings to becomes an excuse to consume food; that is how the habit of compulsive overeating during moments of emotional crisis develop, and before long you ate just to eat and /or because of a feeling, not because you are/were hungry, it becomes a negative ingrained habit that is developed over time; this is not good for many reasons; but specifically your aiding into contributing to major health problems, and it doesn't change the activating situation, nor

2

does this behavior increase a sense of well-being. This is self defeating behavior, STOP IT!!

Recognizing Negative Cognition: *(Thinking, self-talk)* If your sad , broken hearted, and/or depressed, you will have a difficult time managing most of your other life areas, so the process of the self talk is vital to assist with motivation, building self esteem, and encouragement to keep on going and trying.

REACHING WITHIN
(Carmella Irick)

When I reflect on me what do I see? Am I looking at me with a clear heart, and eyes to see, or do I see that disruptive image of me, I must Reach Within.

Reaching Within; when I can see me in my entire splendor, and glory that the creator of the universe, has bestowed unto me all my wonderful qualities, and yes my beauty, I am beautifully made, unique for there is only one of me. I must remember that.

My beauty you see is expressed in many ways, can't you see it? I do its when I say hello, can I help you. I am so wonderful, its manifest itself when I cook a meal I cook with so much love, devotion, and yes passion too.

Once again I tell you, and I tell me, my beauty is within for you see my friend what you see is what you get, it is not in a package its deep within. The soul of a person the heart you see, if you take the time to really look at me you will see that I am magnificent, voluptuous, warm, and kind-hearted; the core of a woman, a real human being.

Reaching Within; I must always seek inner love and peace for I am wonderfully made my creator loves me more than I can image, so I must seek sanctuary in the creator when I feel down, sad, and yes broken heated, by words and oh those sarcastic looks I get from time to time.

I am divine, dynamic, sensual, erotic, full of love, energy, and a zest for life, for I am simply a wonderful creation sent here from the creator to contribute my piece to the world, what that may entail I do not know; but I do know that I must reach within, and realize that I am simply wonderful,

3

and that this is my temple, my body, my holy place where the creator dwells, so I must take care of it, and always be willing to reach within. *(Author Carmella I)*

When we talk about holistic health and/or care as a health care provider we mean; wellness approaches that addresses the body, mind and spirit or the physical, emotional and spiritual aspects of an individual. A holistic health approach views the body, mind and spirit as one entity they are intertwined. What affects one affects the others. Let's examine the body as a machine, you need food fuel to make the body GO the body needs energy to move, and repair it's self, and your brain needs it to function. Stress/emotions plays a major part in interrupting homeostasis *(Balance: The body is constantly seeking to maintain this harmony state to function properly period, if the body is not in sync there will be illness. whether physical or emotional.*

Food Maintenance is designed with the holistic approach in mind, by making the connection, by understanding that you have the power and ability to change yourself, by taking a proactive approach; in regards to how you enhance your living, and eating habits. Food Maintenance encompasses a cognitive and behavioral approach related to you; stress, anger, frustration, ect. Play a major role in the negative eating patterns; however, through FM you will learn to recognize the negative behaviors by self exploration, and learning to embrace all of you, and maybe develop and/or enhance a since of spirituality, i.e. the cosmos or universe, focusing on your positive energy, what ever that may mean to you.

The Self-healing is a phrase applied to the process of recovery (generally from psychological disturbances, trauma, etc.), motivated by and directed by the individual. The value of self-healing lies in its ability to be tailored to the unique experience and requirements of the individual. The process can be helped and accelerated with introspection techniques such as **Meditation**, herbal, and spiritual/spirituality. Holistic health is not itself a method of treatment, but is an approach to how treatment should be applied. Holistic concepts of **health** and **fitness** view achieving and maintaining good health as requiring more than just taking care of the various singular components that make up the physical body, additionally incorporating aspects such as **emotional** and **spiritual** well-being. The goal is a wellness that encompasses the entire person. When symptoms develop, it is often long after the cause of the symptoms occurred; the holistic approach focuses on the root cause.

I am losing weight for me, because I love me. My decision to lose weight is a choice, not an obligation. I am choosing to make my well being a priority. I have made this choice because I care about myself. No one is forcing this decision on me and I can stop at any time - but I choose to continue because I am looking forward to the reward of a slimmer and more energized me. I do not see my weight loss plan as deprivation. I view it as an investment that I know will lead to greater good, to a level of satisfaction with my life and myself that food can never give me. I am choosing to fill my body with good foods that promote a healthy life. I am choosing to make time to exercise. I make these choices because I know they are what I need to be healthy and whole. I treat myself as kindly as I would a cherished friend. If I invite a dear friend into my home, I do not serve her junk and neither do I deny her the healthy food she needs to feel nourished and satisfied. The food I set in front of her is prepared out of love and a desire for her contentment. I treat myself with the same amount of consideration and respect, planning, cooking and eating as my own honored guest.

Helene Lerner states that in the emotional dimension a compulsive eater is not "eating down" feelings, but rather expressing the "inner hunger."

Self-Reflection Questions:
1. Do I see my weight loss as a choice or an obligation?
2. In what ways do I honor my body?
3. In what ways do I need to improve the way I treat my body?
   http://www.acqyr.com

Exercise is a daily routine in my life. Just as waking, eating, and drinking are a daily part of my life, exercise is too. I have a daily routine of things that are good for me such as eating healthy and getting a generous amount of sleep and especially, exercising my body. I do these things to take care of myself and I do them because they are a part of my daily self-care, and self love practices. It is important to have a routine. Having a schedule brings me balance and helps my body in all its functions. Just as waking in the morning, eating breakfast, showering, brushing my teeth and getting dressed are a part of my daily routine; exercise too is a part of that routine. I establish clarity and vitality by making exercise a part of my schedule.

For the purpose of this book I choose to utilize the Ayurveda, holistic model for wellness; simply for its simplicity, and well defined balance/harmony. Ayurveda traces its origins to the Vedas the Atharvaveda in particular, and is connected to religion and mythology. The Sushruta Samhita of Sushruta appeared during the 1st millennium BC Dwivedi & Dwivedi (2007)

Ayurveda ; the 'science of life') is a system of traditional medicine native to India, and practiced in other parts of the world as a form of alternative medicine. In Sanskrit, the word Ayurveda comprises the words yus, meaning 'life' and veda, meaning 'science'. Evolving throughout its history, Ayurveda remains an influential system of medicine in South Asia Chopra (2003)

Include in this section is the Ayurvedic Mind, Body Quiz, So that you can discover your Mind Body Type, Reprinted from (Chopra Deepak 2001).

Ayurveda believes in 'five great elements' (earth, water, fire, air and space) forming the universe, including the human body Blood, flesh, fat, bone, marrow, chyle, and semen are believed to be the seven primary constituent elements of the body. Ayurveda stresses a balance of three substances: wind/spirit/air, phlegm, and bile, each representing divine forces. Chopra (2003)

According to Ayurvedic beliefs, the doctrine of these three Dosas VATA (wind/spirit/air), PITTA (bile) and KAPHA (phlegm) is important.

Traditional beliefs hold that humans possess a unique constellation of Dosas.Underwood & Rhodes (2008). It is believed that building a healthy metabolic system, attaining good digestion, and proper excretion leads to vitality. Ayurveda also focuses on exercise, yoga, meditation. Chopra (2003)

Beginning the process of self-healing, and self help it is imperative to find out why you are overeating, and let's work on that while we focus on you losing and maintaining your healthy weight/status. Include in this section is the Ayurvedic Mind, Body Quiz, So that you can discover your Mind Body Type. The following quiz is divided into three sections.

The first 20 questions , apply to Vata dosha, the second section applies to the Pitta dosha, the third section applies to Kapha dosha, read each question and mark a 0-6 whether it applies to you or not. At the end of each section write down your total score and compare the three sections these will determine your body type.

0=dose not apply
3=Applies to me somewhat (or some of the time)
6-Applies to me mostly (or nearly all the time)

How to determine your body type:
- If one dosha score is much higher than the others, you're probably a single-dosha type.
- If no single dosha score dominated you are a two- dosha type
- If your three dosha score are nearly equal you may be a three- dosha type

CHARACTERTISTICS VATA: Vata is always in motion, always shifting reversing direction. Vata types are more variable than pitta, Kaphas, and their behavior from day to day is difficult to predict. Burst of energy, both mental & physical, appear suddenly, & then vanish just as quickly. Vata are consistently inconsistent. This is present in their digestion, moods, emotions, and the state of their general health, they are particularly vulnerable to minor illnesses colds and flu.

Characteristics of Vata Type:
- Light, thin build Performs activity quickly
- Irregular hunger and digestion, Tendency to worry
- Light, interrupted sleep; tendency toward insomnia
- Enthusiasm, vivaciousness, imagination

- Quick to grasp new information, also quick to forget.
- Tendency to be constipated
- Tires easily, tendency to overexert
- Mental/physical energy comes in bursts.

It is very Vata to:
- Be hungry at any time of the day or night
- Love excitement and constant change
- Go to sleep at different times every night, skips meals general irregular habits
- Digest food well one day & poorly the next.
- Walks quickly
- Displays bursts of emotions that are short-lived and quickly forgotten.

CHARACTERTISTICS PITTA: Pitta is intensity association with the heart is evident even in physical characteristics of Pitta types, Pitta are ambitious driven individuals with bold styles of self-expression and tendency to become argumentative if challenged. Balance Pitta are affectionate. Only when stress, improper diet, other destabilizing influences come into play does the aggressive, critical side of Pitta nature begins

Characteristics of Pitta Type:
- Medium build, Cannot skip a meal
- Medium strength and endurance
- Sharp hunger and thirst, strong digestion
- Aversion to sun, & hot weather.
- Enterprising personality, sharp intellect, likes challenges. Precise, articulate, speech

It is very Pitta to:
- Feels ravenous if dinner is half-I hour late.
- Lives by a watch, resents have time wasted.
- Takes command of situations or feel that you should.
- Walks with determined stride.
- Learn from experience that others sometimes find to demanding or critical.

CHARACTERTISTICS KAPHA: Is the calmest, most stable dosha, & Kapha goes out of balance less easily than Vata, Pitta, Kapha brings structure, stamina to the physiology, & these characteristics are evident in the stocky build of many kapha types, By nature Kaphas are serene & optimistic, slow to anger, & prefer to consider all points of view before taking a position, when out of balance, kaphas can be lethargic, indecisive. Benefit from vigorous exercise, diet that counters their natural tendency toward overweight. Kapha are; naturally loving and considerate, their innate strength providesprotection against illness.

Characteristics of Kapha Type:
- Solid, powerful build; excellent physical strength and endurance. Steady energy; slow and graceful in action Tranquil, relaxed personality; slow to anger. Cool, smooth thick, pale, often oily skin.
- Slow to grasp new information, but good retention memory.
- Heavy, prolonged sleep. Tendency toward overweight. Slow digestion, mild hunger.
- Affectionate, tolerant, forgiving. Tendency to be possessive and complacent.

It is very Kapha to:
- Mull things over for a long time before making a decision.
- Wake up slowly, lie in bed for a long time, and need coffee upon arising.
- Be happy with the status quo and preserve it by conciliating others. Respect other's feelings and feel genuine empathy
- Seek emotional comfort from eating.

Ayurvedic Mind, Body Quiz

SECTION 1 VITA

		Does not Apply		Applies sometimes			Applies most time	
1.	I perform activities very quickly	0	1	2	3	4	5	6
2.	I am not good at memorizing things and then remembering them later	0	1	2	3	4	5	6
3.	I am enthusiastic and vivacious by nature.	0	1	2	3	4	5	6
4.	I have a thin physique, I don't gain weight easily.	0	1	2	3	4	5	6
5.	I have always learned new things very quickly.	0	1	2	3	4	5	6
6.	My movement while walking is light and quick.	0	1	2	3	4	5	6
7.	I tend to have difficulty making decisions.	0	1	2	3	4	5	6
8.	I tend to develop gas and become constipated easily.	0	1	2	3	4	5	6
9.	I tend to have cold hands and feet.	0	1	2	3	4	5	6
10.	I become anxious or worried frequently	0	1	2	3	4	5	6
11.	I don't tolerate cold weather as well as most people do.	0	1	2	3	4	5	6
12.	I speak quickly and my friends think that I'm talkative.	0	1	2	3	4	5	6
13.	My mood changes easily and I am somewhat emotional by nature.	0	1	2	3	4	5	6
14.	I often have difficulty falling asleep or having a sound night sleep.	0	1	2	3	4	5	6
15.	My skin tend to be very dry, especially in winter	0	1	2	3	4	5	6
16.	My mind is very active sometimes restless, but also very imaginative.	0	1	2	3	4	5	6
17.	My movements are quick and active; my energy tends to come in bursts.	0	1	2	3	4	5	6
18.	I am easily excitable.	0	1	2	3	4	5	6
19.	I tend to be irregular in my eating and sleeping habits.	0	1	2	3	4	5	6
20.	I learn quickly, but I forget quickly	0	1	2	3	4	5	6

SECTION 2 PITA

		Does not Apply		Applies sometimes			Applies most time	
1.	I consider myself to be very efficient.	0	1	2	3	4	5	6
2.	In my activities, I try to be extremely precise and orderly.	0	1	2	3	4	5	6
3.	I am strong-minded and have a somewhat forced manner.	0	1	2	3	4	5	6
4.	I feel uncomfortable or become easily fatigued in hot weather more than others	0	1	2	3	4	5	6
5.	I tend to perspire easily.	0	1	2	3	4	5	6
6.	Even through I might not always show it, I become irritable or angry quite easily.	0	1	2	3	4	5	6
7.	If I skip or delay a meal I become uncomfortable.	0	1	2	3	4	5	6
8.	One or more of the following characteristics, Describes my hair: thin, fine, straight, course early graying, balding, red, blond, brown, and black.	0	1	2	3	4	5	6
9.	I have a strong appetite; if I want to, I can eat a lot.	0	1	2	3	4	5	6
10.	Many people consider me stubborn.	0	1	2	3	4	5	6
11.	I am very regular in my bowel habits; it is more Common for me to have loose stools than constipation.	0	1	2	3	4	5	6
12.	I become inpatient easily.	0	1	2	3	4	5	6
13.	I tend to be a perfectionist about details.	0	1	2	3	4	5	6
14.	I get angry quite easily, but then I quickly forget about it.	0	1	2	3	4	5	6
15.	I am very found of cold foods, such as ice cream, and ice cold drinks	0	1	2	3	4	5	6
16.	I am more likely to feel that a room is too hot than to cold	0	1	2	3	4	5	6
17.	I don't tolerate foods that are very hot & spicy.	0	1	2	3	4	5	6
18.	I am not as tolerant of disagreements as I should be.	0	1	2	3	4	5	6
19.	I tend to be quite critical of others and also of myself.	0	1	2	3	4	5	6
20.	I enjoy challenges, and when I want something, I am Very determined in my efforts to get it.	0	1	2	3	4	5	6

SECTION 3 KAPHA

		Does not Apply		Applies sometimes		Applies most time		
1.	My natural tendency is to do things in a slow and relaxed fashion.	0	1	2	3	4	5	6
2.	I gain weight more easily than most people And lose it more slowly.	0	1	2	3	4	5	6
3.	I have a placid and calm disposition, I'm not easily ruffled.	0	1	2	3	4	5	6
4.	I can skip meals easily without any significant discomfort.	0	1	2	3	4	5	6
5.	I have a tendency toward excess mucus or Phlegm, chronic congestion, asthma, sinuses	0	1	2	3	4	5	6
6.	I must get at least 8 hours of sleep to be comfortable the next day.	0	1	2	3	4	5	6
7.	I sleep very deeply.	0	1	2	3	4	5	6
8.	I am calm by nature and not easily angered.	0	1	2	3	4	5	6
9.	I don't learn as quickly as some people, but I have excellent retention and long memory.	0	1	2	3	4	5	6
10.	I have a tendency toward becoming plump, Store extra fat easily.	0	1	2	3	4	5	6
11.	Weather that is cool and damp bothers me.	0	1	2	3	4	5	6
12.	My hair is thick dark, and wavy.	0	1	2	3	4	5	6
13.	I have smooth, soft skin with pale complexion	0	1	2	3	4	5	6
14.	I have a large, solid body build.	0	1	2	3	4	5	6
15.	The following word describe me well; serene, sweet-natured, affectionate, forgiving	0	1	2	3	4	5	6
16.	I have a slow digestion, which makes me feel heavy after eating	0	1	2	3	4	5	6
17.	I have very good stamina and physical endurance As well as a steady level of energy.	0	1	2	3	4	5	6
18.	I general walk with a slow measure gait.	0	1	2	3	4	5	6
19.	I'm a slow eater and am slow methodical in my action	0	1	2	3	4	5	6
20.	I have a tendency toward oversleeping and Grogginess upon awakening and am general slow To get up in the morning.	0	1	2	3	4	5	6

Chapter Two
Basic Nutrition & Medical Facts

Abbreviations Used:

BMI – Body mass index.
CI – Confidence interval.
NCHS – National Center for Health Statistics
NH – non-Hispanic
NHANES – National Health and Nutrition Examination Survey, NCHS
NHES – National Health Examination Survey, NCHS
NHIS – National Health Interview Survey, NCHS
FM- Food Maintenance

****

You must have food to sustain life however when the vast majority of society is overweight obese, simple by choosing to eat with an unhealthy attitude and/or perspective in relationship to food you are what you eat, nutrition is vital in maintain balance, harmony/balance. Nutrition is a basic fundamental need that must be met by all persons for the sole benefit of sustaining life, in order to promote growth, health and wellness to maintain energy to function also to prevent disease. **The four basic** nutrients needed for growth and health **are Water,** Carbohydrates, Proteins, and Fats these are the basic building blocks of a good diet. By choosing the healthiest forms of each of these nutrients, and eating them in the proper balance, you enable your body to function at its optimal level. Holistic concepts of health and fitness view achieving and maintaining good health, requiring more than just taking care of a singular components that make up the physical body, by incorporating aspects such as emotional and spiritual well-being, in addition too physical exercise specific to toning and strengthening muscle..

Water: The human body is two-thirds water. Water is an essential nutrient that is involved in every function of the body.

Carbohydrates: Carbohydrates supply the body with the energy it needs to function. They are found almost exclusively in plant foods, such as fruits, vegetables, peas, and beans.

Fats: Although much attention has been focused on the need to reduce dietary fat, the body does need fat, to provide concentrated source of a stored form of energy; also protects internal organs and maintains body temperature.

Protein: Protein is essential for growth and development, provides energy for the body. Protein builds and repairs body tissues, produces antibodies to fight off disease, facilitates with energy to burn calories

Fiber: Fiber is the part of a plant that is resistant to the body's digestive enzymes. Fiber speeds the movement of undigested materials through the intestine. Additional note for those that express a desire to participate in a vegetarian Food Maintenance philosophy Protein and fiber consumption must be increased by consuming a variety of vegetables, whole grain, ands nuts.

Vitamins: Facilitate metabolism of proteins, fats, and Carbohydrates: promote life and growth processes; maintains and regulate body functions. Important note ladies, Vitamin-C promotes optimal absorption of Iron.

Carbohydrates: Carbohydrates supply the body with the energy it needs to function. They are found almost exclusively in plant foods, such as fruits, vegetables, peas, and beans. Milk and milk products are the only foods derived from animals that contain a significant amount of carbohydrates. It is recommended that about 60 percent of your total daily calories come from carbohydrates. Carbohydrates are divided into two groups—simple carbohydrates and complex carbohydrates.

Dietary Suggestions

Eat a Meal High in Carbohydrates: Good sources of carbohydrates include rice, pasta, potatoes, breads, air-popped popcorn and low-cal cookies.

Eat Food High in Fiber: Eat more fiber to keep your digestive system moving. Your meals should provide at least 25 grams of fiber per day. Fruits, vegetables, and grains are excellent sources of fiber. For breakfast, eat whole fruits instead of just juice, whole-grain cereals, and fiber-fortified muffins.

Chapter Three
Medical Facts

Here are some facts you need to know. These medical conditions are related to obesity and being overweight, and all medical facts are cited according to their sources. Included are some statistics and women's heart health. This is just a basic overview of some medical facts. I encourage you to regularly visit your primary physician for check-ups and mammograms, especially women of color,

Hypertension (High Blood Pressure): High blood pressure is a rather unique condition because, unlike most diseases, it has no identifying symptoms. For this reason, blood pressure is commonly referred to as *the silent killer* and generally defined as a reading of 140/90 or greater recorded on at least three separate occasions. Both the systolic and diastolic blood pressure are important determinants of cardiovascular risk, so both are used in evaluating overall blood pressure status. For most people, the first time they discover their high blood pressure is during a routine visit to their doctor's office for an unrelated complaint or a regularly scheduled health maintenance appointment. (Source: www.about.com)

Diabetes and high blood pressure commonly occur together, and the combination is known to be more dangerous than either disease by itself. Understanding why these two diseases so often occur in the same patients has been a decades long undertaking of the medical and scientific communities. While there are still many details to uncover, much is known about the factors that lead to these diseases. (Source: www.about.com)

Diabetes Type 1: Diabetes, formerly called juvenile diabetes or insulin-dependent diabetes, is usually first diagnosed in children, teenagers, or young adults. In this form of diabetes, the beta cells of the pancreas no longer make insulin because the body's immune system has attacked and destroyed them. Treatment for Type 1 diabetes includes taking insulin shots or using an insulin pump, making wise food choices, exercising regularly, taking aspirin daily (for some), and controlling blood pressure and cholesterol. (Source: www.about.com)

Diabetes Type 2: Diabetes, formerly called adult-onset or non insulin-dependent diabetes, is the most common form of diabetes. People can develop Type 2 diabetes at any age, even during childhood. This form of diabetes usually begins with insulin resistance, a condition in which fat, muscle, and liver cells do not use insulin properly. At first, the pancreas keeps up with the added demand by producing more insulin. In time, however, it loses the ability to secrete enough insulin in response to meals. Being overweight and inactive increases the chances of developing Type 2 diabetes. Treatment includes taking diabetes medicines, making wise food choices, exercising regularly, taking aspirin daily, and controlling blood pressure and cholesterol. (Source: www.about.com)

Gestational Diabetes: Some women develop gestational diabetes during the late stages of pregnancy. Although this form of diabetes usually goes away after the baby is born, a woman who has had it is more likely to develop Type 2 diabetes later in life. Gestational diabetes is caused by the hormones of pregnancy or a shortage of insulin. Another common time for diagnosis is during a woman's first prenatal visit during pregnancy. Since most first time mothers tend to be young, regular visits to the doctor aren't a priority until they become pregnant, leading to an uncharacteristically high rate of diagnosis in this patient population. (Source: www.about.com)

(CVA) Stoke: Sudden loss of consciousness followed by paralysis, caused by bleeding into the brain, formation of a blood clot causing blockage and/or rupture of an artery in the brain resulting in bleeding into the subarachnoid space. Chronic health conditions such as high blood pressure and diabetes can increase your risk, as well as lifestyle choices such as smoking cigarettes, being overweight, or drinking excessively. Men, African-Americans, and people with a family history of stroke have a higher risk as well. If you have already had a stroke or a transient ischemic attack (referred to as a TIA or *mini-stroke*), you are at the highest risk. Warning signs include sudden unexplained numbness or tingling (especially on one side), slurred speech, blurred vision, stumbling, or clumsiness. **(Source:** www.about.com)

Cholesterol Facts: Protect your heart by lowering cholesterol. Cholesterol levels are checked by a blood test and should be a routine part of your annual checkup. If you have high cholesterol, your doctor may decide to check it more often. Your cholesterol level should be in the range of 140 to 200 milligrams of cholesterol, per deciliter of blood. People who have high cholesterol are at higher risk of heart attack and stroke. Cholesterol levels that are too low can be an indication of health problems such as liver cancer. The type of cholesterol that is found can also make a difference to your health risk. LDL or low-density lipoproteins are considered bad" cholesterol while HDL or high-density lipoproteins are considered good cholesterol. Your risk of heart disease will be lower if your HDL accounts for more than 25% of your total cholesterol. (Source: www.about.com)

Heart Attacks: Women's Guide to Heart Health. There is little equality between the sexes in heart attack symptoms. If you ask most women over the age of 50 what they think is the greatest threat to their health and life, most will mistakenly answer cancer. Over the last few years cancer, specifically breast, uterine and ovarian cancers, have been in the spotlight as women's biggest health concern. However, women face an even greater threat from heart disease. Heart disease and heart attacks claim the lives of more American women than men each year, and pose a greater threat to American women than all forms of cancer combined. While most women can tell you the *classic*" symptoms of heart attack most do not realize that a woman's symptoms can be very different. This may significantly delay life saving treatment. It is a well-documented fact that prompts recognition, and treatment of heart attack can save lives. Dr. Bairey Merz of Cedars-Sinai Medical Center offers the following heart tips that are especially for women:

1. If you're over age 18, have your blood pressure checked annually; over age 45, have your blood cholesterol and blood sugar checked each year; and if you have a family history of heart disease in a relative prior to the age of 60, especially in a female relative, ask your physician to do these tests at earlier ages and to consider additional tests such as treadmill testing and other heart disease screening tests.

2. Be aware that the symptoms for women having a heart attack are often different from those of a man, but any of the following symptoms can occur in men and women:

CLASSIC SYMPTOMS
1. Squeezing Chest Pain
2. Shortness of Breath
3. Sweating
4. Discomfort/Pain Between Shoulder Blades
5. Pain Spreading to Shoulders, Neck, or Arm

MORE LIKELY IN WOMEN
1. Indigestion or Gas-like Pain
2. Dizziness, Nausea, or Vomiting
3. Unexplained Weakness, Fatigue
4. Tightness in Chest
5. Recurring Chest Discomfort
6. Sense of Impending Doom
(Source: www.about.com)

An Important Message for Women:

According to Women's Heart Foundation, heart disease is the number one killer of American women. Recognizing symptoms and risks, making lifestyle changes, and getting timely care can save a woman's life. Interestingly, according to disease reports from the New York Department of Health and the 2004 Women's Heart Day Program in Manhattan, while diabetes rates are soaring around the country, the incidence of diabetes in lower Manhattan is going down. Why? The average New Yorker walks four miles a day! *Take Care of Your Heart©. http://www.womensheart.org*

Statistics on Overweight Adults/Children and Reported Activity Levels
Less than one-third (31.8 percent) of U.S. adults get regular leisure-time physical activity (defined as light or moderate activity five times or more per week for 30 minutes or more each time and/or vigorous activity three times or more per week for 20 minutes or more each time). About 10 percent of adults do no physical activity at all in their leisure time.

Nearly two-thirds of U.S. adults are overweight (BMI > 25, which includes those who are obese). All adults (20+ years old): 129.6 million (64.5 percent), Women (20+ years old): 64.5 million (61.9 percent), Men (20+ years old): 65.1 million (67.2 percent). Nearly one-third of U.S. adults are obese (BMI > 30). All adults (20+ years old): 61.3 million (30.5 percent), Women (20+ years old): 34.7 million (33.4 percent), Men (20+ years old): 26.6 million (27.5 percent).

Take it one step at a time. It takes time to build new healthy habits. Follow along each day to walk, exercise, eat right, set and achieve goals—and have some fun along the way. There are many activity-based programs out-lined herein with support documents, downloads, and website links. All rep-resent a CALL TO ACTION to be more active to prevent early death from heart disease. It's time for families to get involved. Take action. Be fit. *Take Care of Your Heart©. http://www.womensheart.org*

Associated Conditions for Overweight and Obesity
According to wrongdiagnosis.com, the medical facts listed in this section show conditions that are regarded as associated with diabetes. These include:

Heart Disease: The leading cause of death for both men and women in the United States. Heart disease includes heart attack, heart failure, and *angina* (chest pain caused by reduced blood flow to the heart). (Source: www.wrongdiagnoisis.com)

Stroke: A stroke is sometimes called a *brain attack*. Most strokes are caused by a blood clot blocking an artery that takes blood to the brain. (Source: www.wrongdiagnoisis.com)

17

Diabetes: Overweight people are twice as likely to develop Type 2 diabetes as people who are not overweight. Type 2 diabetes reduces your body's ability to control your blood sugar. It is a major cause of early death, heart disease, kidney disease, stroke, and blindness. (Source: www.wrongdiagnoisis.com)

Cancer: Cancer of the gallbladder, breast, uterus, cervix, and ovaries (for women). Overweight men are at greater risk for developing cancer of the colon, rectum, and prostate. (Source: www.wrongdiagnoisis.com)

Gallstones or Gallbladder Disease: Gallbladder disease and gallstones are more common if you are overweight. Your risk of disease increases as your weight increases. However, weight loss itself, particularly rapid weight loss or loss of a large amount of weight, can actually increase your chances of getting gallstones. Modest, slow weight loss of about 1 pound a week is less likely to cause gallstones. (Source: www.wrongdiagnoisis.com

Osteoarthritis (wearing away of the joints): Osteoarthritis is a common joint disorder that most often affects the joints in your knees, hips, and lower back. Extra weight puts extra pressure on these joints and wears away the cartilage (tissue that cushions the joints) that normally protects them. Weight loss may improve the symptoms of osteoarthritis. (Source: www.wrongdiagnoisis.com

Gout (joint pain caused by excess *uric acid*): Gout is a joint disease caused by high levels of uric acid in the blood. Uric acid sometimes forms crystals that are deposited in the joints. Gout is more common in overweight people. If you have a history of gout, check with your doctor before trying to lose weight. Some diets may lead to an attack of gout in people who have high levels of uric acid or who have had gout before. (Source: www.wrongdiagnoisis.com)

Breathing Problems: Breathing problems, including sleep apnea (interrupted breathing during sleep). Sleep apnea is a serious condition that can cause a person to stop breathing for short periods during sleep and to snore heavily. Sleep apnea may cause daytime sleepiness and even heart failure. The risk for sleep apnea increases with higher body weights. Weight loss usually improves sleep apnea. (Source: www.wrongdiagnoisis.com)

High Blood Cholesterol: High levels of total cholesterol, LDL cholesterol (bad cholesterol) and *triglycerides* (another type of fat in the blood) can lead to heart disease. Obesity is also linked to low levels of HDL cholesterol (good cholesterol). Weight loss can improve your cholesterol levels. (Source: www.wrongdiagnoisis.com

High Blood Pressure: High blood pressure is a major risk factor for heart disease and stroke. Obese adults are twice as likely to have high blood pressure as those who are at a healthy weight. Weight loss can lower your blood pressure. (Source: www.wrongdiagnoisis.com

Complications of Pregnancy: Obesity increases the risks of high blood pressure and a type of diabetes that develops during pregnancy. Obese women are more likely to have problems with labor and delivery. (Source: www.wrongdiagnoisis.com

Irregular Menstrual Cycles and Infertility: Abdominal obesity is linked to *polycystic ovary syndrome*, a cause of infertility in women. (Source: www.wrongdiagnoisis.com. Original excerpt from Obesity: NWHIC)

Psychological and Social Effects, Such as Depression and Discrimination: One of the most painful aspects of obesity may be the emotional suffering it causes. American society places great emphasis on physical appearance, equating attractiveness with slimness, especially in women. Feelings of rejection, shame, or depression are common. (Source: www.wrongdiagnoisis.com. Original excerpt from Obesity: NWHIC)

Included is a list of Associated Medical Conditions Mentioned by Various Sources as Associated with Overweight Includes:

- Type 2 diabetes
- Heart disease
- Stroke
- Hypertension - 23.9% of overweight men and 23.0% of overweight women have hypertension
- Gallbladder disease
- Osteoarthritis
- Breathing difficulties
- Uterine cancer
- Breast cancer
- Colorectal cancer
- Kidney cancer
- Gallbladder cancer
- Sleep apnea

Another Type of Associated Condition Is One for which Overweight Is Itself a Risk Factor

- Cardiovascular Disease
- Colorectal cancer
- Coronary heart disease
- Deep vein thrombosis

- Gastroesophageal Reflux Disease
- Gout
- Heart attack
- Heart disease
- Heart failure
- High Cholesterol
- Hypertension
- Obstructive sleep apnea
- Osteoarthritis
- Proteinuria
- Pulmonary embolism
- Sleep apnea
- Slipped epiphysis
- Snoring
- Superficial Thrombophlebitis
- Thrombosis
- Uterine Cancer

http://www.wrongdiagnosis.com/o/overweight/stats.htm

Overweight and Obesity Statistics: Data from the CDC's YRBS 2005 survey showed that the prevalence of being overweight was higher among non-Hispanic black (16.0%) and Hispanic (16.8%) than non-Hispanic white (11.8%) students; higher among non-Hispanic black female (16.1%) and Hispanic female (12.1%) than non-Hispanic white female (8.2%) students; and higher among non-Hispanic black male (15.9%) and Hispanic male (21.3%) than non-Hispanic white male (15.2%) students. The prevalence of being at risk for being overweight was higher among non-Hispanic black (19.8%) and Hispanic (16.7%) than non-Hispanic white (14.5%) students; higher among non-Hispanic black female (22.6%) than non-Hispanic white female (13.8%) and Hispanic female (16.8%) students; and higher among Hispanic male (16.5%) and non-Hispanic black male (16.7%) than non-Hispanic white male (15.2%) students. (Source: 2008, American Heart Association, www.americanheart.org. Original Source: MMWR Surveill Summ. 2006;55:1-108.).

This was the most current data I could find during the writing of this book; it is my sincere desire to increase your awareness about this medical epidemic that is affecting women and children throughout the USA, and the urgent need for changing our eating behaviors, especially women of color. It is noted in countless medical publications that low income persons are hit the hardest due to the lack of adequate healthcare services and the economic status. It is a know fact that women who are pregnant and on food stamps are at greater risk for nutritional deficiencies. I encourage you all to make the time for yourself and practice self-care.

Chapter Four
Taking Back Your Power and Control by Taking Action

Changing Our Self-concept and Building Self-esteem
Based on the holistic approach and philosophy of FM, the five unifying concepts; fosters the focus of working from the inside out developing a sense of self worth and self esteem. Will allow each individual to internalize and utilize this information for their specific areas of need/enhancement. Once again as stated earlier change is internal. I have found internal self-esteem building, to be very beneficial to others and myself, I have utilized self-esteem building as one of the major core concepts in practices. I believe that what I teach; gives me a sense of well-being, increases my self esteem and gives me creditably among the persons I service. Working in the field of addictions and nursing I have found that when persons are in a state of un-wellness this can have a dramatic impact on an individuals confidences, sense of self, and slows down the healing process. And being overweight and/or lacking impulse control over any substances i.e. food, alcohol; ect, the negative psychological effects can causes sever and/or detrimental emotional harm, stress, and potential periods of mild to serve depression. *(As stated through out this self-help book; If at any point that you come to realize that you may need additional services pleased see a physician, and as always before you start any modifications in diet and physical activity seek out medical advice from a medical provider).* Change starts when you decide that you are willing to work on your deficit life areas.

This section is devoted to your self-concept and to build your self-esteem and, as a result, enables you to be happier and to achieve more of your desired potential, to be all that you can be. The goal isn't to just accept yourself, in your present state of being regardless of how you are behaving; this behavior can be changed or modified. *"I will strive to be better than I was yesterday, and what did I learn from yesterday to take into today" (Author)*

Working in the field of addictions and nursing, I have found that when people are in a state of unwellness, this has a dramatic impact on an individual's confidence, sense of self, and slows down the healing process. In addition, being overweight and/or lacking impulse control over any substances, i.e., food, alcohol, etc., the negative psychological effects can cause severe and/or detrimental emotional harm, stress, and potential periods of mild to severe depression. *(As stated throughout this self-help book, if at any point you come to realize that you may need additional services, please see a physician and, as always, before you start any modifications in diet and physical activity, seek out medical advice from a medical provider.)* Change starts when you decide that you are willing to work on your deficit life areas.

This section is devoted to your self-concept, to build your self-esteem, and, as a result, enable you to be happier and to achieve more of your desired potential; to be all that you can be. The goal isn't to just accept yourself in your present state of being regardless of how you are behaving; this behavior can be changed or modified. *"I will strive to be better than I was yesterday, and what did I learn from yesterday to take into today" (Author)*

The fact remains diets don't work because you are either depriving yourself of food and/or using food to fill a void in your life. The main problem with that is, no matter where you go, you take you with you, while carrying the same problem(s), and then the vicious cycle begins. You know, the ups and downs that cause your self-esteem to crash once again and you say, *"I failed." No you didn't fail you just didn't maintain the weight, and you never took the time to examine the root cause.*

Well, let's get healthy and examine self, in order to begin learning better eating habits for a healthier you and long-term eating discipline.

> *"We are what we think. All that we are arises with our thoughts. With our thoughts, we make the world." The Buddha*

The definition of self-esteem: **"appreciating my own worth** and importance, and having the character to **be accountable** for myself and to **act responsibly."** *Self-esteem is self-love, responsibility, and respect for my present self and my future self; yesterday happened but I have today (Unknown).*

Purposes
- To have a more positive self-concept.
- To see yourself honestly and to like or at least accept yourself.
- To remove the internal barriers keeping you from doing your best.

Several researchers suggest that humans are best understood by accepting that we have many selves. For instance, we are not only aware of many current traits, but we have selves leftover from the past (our *former* selves) and we have **potential future selves**, such as *hoped for selves*, *ideal* selves, *successful* selves, and also *feared selves*, *incompetent* selves, etc. Most of us only consider the *current* selves, neglecting the *future* and *past* selves, although what you want to become and what you fear becoming powerfully affect your behavior. All the*se internal* -ideas, memory, imagery, hopes, and self-evaluation—is complexly intertwined with simple behavior, motivation. However, for clarity and the progression of this book, I want to focus on getting you to think about why you use food, and in this process of self-awareness, if you find that you need additional services, please seek what you need to become, evolve, and transform.

To discuss the concepts of "Self" you must begin to reflect on your life experiences from childhood, *(family of origin)*,adolescence,*(initial developing self)* into adult hood, *(present state of being) your* potential self *(the hoped for and future goals/dreams desires wants)*, Fears and feeling inferior may sometimes compel us to work very hard to succeed. Most of the time, however, failure makes us feel incompetent and uninterested in the task (Kohn, 1994) *Fear* of the unknown affect your, thoughts and behaviors, fear can cause you to doubt your abilities that you have inside of yourself However, for clarity, and this book I want to focus on getting you to begin to think about why you use food, and in this process of self awareness if you find that you need additional services please seek what you need to become, evolve, transform. For some pain is a motivator, pain will cause an individual to make the necessary needed changes in his/her life. Self reflection cause each unique individual to look at self in a holistic manner childhood where you come from, adolescence, adapting, modeling developing your sense of self, style, ect,.. adulthood/ present here and now, your potential self where are you going, or where do you see yourself, self reflection allows you to understand how each life step has contributed to your current beliefs, and way of responding to others and how and why you may or may not respond or feel based on core values, belief system in addition too learned behaviors along the way i.e. negative eating to seek comfort, over working to avoid family/partner disruptions.

To talk about identity is to talk about the condition character of being oneself Identity defines people and gives meaning to all aspect of their lives. It is shaped by life experiences past and present. "You determine who and what you will become". "Speak yourself into your new existence", tell yourself you can and you will, however you must take some action and responsibility for self. In short, you must know yourself, so you can set your life goals and self actualize. Positive self talk is vital to your emotional success in all areas of your life; you have the ability to do what ever it is you are willing to work at. However, before you can begin the process of making changes to your identity , you must first decide do some self exploration of your identity. FM is about making the mind, body and spirit connection in all aspects of your life, it about being willing to commit to your self for better long-term health, and maintain your desired weight goals, by taking back your personal power and control. And for some this aspects includes a form of or a sence of spirituality.

Spirituality plays a major role in the human condition spirituality presents itself in many forms this varies from person to person, however, as human beings for the most part we seek the calming, loving source of energy, light within self or outside of self. This energy can express, manifest in any form you choose, this is a personal choice.

To the one who feels he/she is an atheist or agnostic; When, I speak to you of God; I mean your own conception of God he/she whatever the you choose, the prospering power of the universe if you so desire.According to Wikipedia online; Spirituality, in a narrow sense, concerns itself with matters of the spirit, a concept closely tied to religious belief and faith, a transcendent reality, and one or more deities. Spiritual matters are thus those matters regarding humankind's ultimate nature and purpose, not only as material biological organisms, but as beings with a unique relationship to that which is perceived to be beyond both time and the material world.

Spirituality may involve perceiving or wishing to perceive life as more important ("higher"), more complex or more integrated with one's world view; as contrasted with the merely sensual. Many spiritual traditions, accordingly, share a common spiritual theme: the "path", "work", practice, or tradition of perceiving and internalizing one's "true" nature and relationship to the rest of existence (God, creation of the universe, or life), and of becoming free of the lesser egoic self (or ego) in favor of being more fully one's "true" "Self".(Wikipedia online)

Changing our self-concept and building self-esteem

Based on the holistic approach and philosophy of FM, concepts; fosters the focus of working from the inside out developing a sense of self worth and self esteem. This will allow each individual to internalize and utilize this information for their specific areas of need/enhancement. Once again as stated earlier change is internal. I have utilized self-esteem building as one of the major core concepts in practices. I believe that what I teach; i must also practice in my daily life, this gives me a sense of well-being, increases my self esteem and gives me creditably among the persons I service. Working in the field of addictions and nursing I have found that when persons are in a state of un-wellness this can have a dramatic impact on an individuals confidences, sense of self, and slows down the healing process. And being overweight and/or lacking impulse control over any substances i.e. food, alcohol; ect, the negative psychological effects can causes sever and/or detrimental emotional harm, stress, and potential periods of mild to serve depression. (*As stated through out this self-help book; If at any point that you come to realize that you may need additional services pleased see a physician, and as always before you start any*

24

modifications in diet and physical activity seek out medical advice from a medical provider). Change starts when you decide that you are willing to work on your life areas.

This section is devoted to your self-concept and to build your self-esteem and, as a result, enables you to be happier and to achieve more of your desired potential, to be all that you can be. The goal isn't to just accept yourself, in your present state of being regardless of how you are behaving; this behavior can be changed or modified. "I will strive to be better than I was yesterday, and what did I learn from yesterday to take into today" (Author)

The fact remains Diet's don't work because you are either depriving yourself of food and/or using food to fill a void in your life; and the main problem with that is, no matter where you go, you take you with you, while carrying all the same problem(s); and then the viscous cycle begins; you know; The up-down, this causes your self esteem to crash once again "I failed". No you didn't fail you just didn't maintain the weight, and you never took the time to examine the root cause. Well let's get healthy and examine self; in order to begin learning better eating habits for a healthier you and long-term eating discipline.

We are what we think. All that we are arises with our thoughts. With our thoughts, we make the world. The Buddha

The definition of self-esteem: favorable opinion of oneself appreciating your self-worth and the importance of your integrity character for your self to practice self-care and self love to respect for my present self and my future self; *Yesterday happen but I have today (Unknown).* The purpose of this section is too

- To appreciate your self increase your self worth
- To see yourself honestly and to accept yourself.
- To remove your personal barriers that keep you from maintaining

To discuss the concepts of "Self" you must begin to reflect on your life experiences from childhood, *(family of origin),*adolescence,*(initial developing self)* into adult hood, *(present state of being) your* potential self *(the hoped for and future goals/dreams desires wants),* Fears and feeling inferior may sometimes compel us to work very hard to succeed. Most of the time, however, failure makes us feel incompetent and uninterested in the task (Kohn, 1994) *Fear of the unknown affect your,* thoughts and behaviors, fear can cause you to doubt your abilities that you have inside of yourself However, for clarity, and this book I want to focus on getting you to begin to think about why you use food, and in this process of self awareness if you find that you need additional services please seek what you need to become, evolve, transform.

For some pain is a motivator, pain will cause an individual to make the necessary needed changes in his/her life. Self reflection cause each unique individual to look at self in a holistic manner childhood where you come from, adolescence, adapting, modeling developing your sense of self, style, ect,.. adulthood/ present here and now, your potential self where are you going, or where do you see yourself, self reflection allows you to understand how each life step has contributed to your current beliefs, and way of responding to others and how and why you may or may not respond or feel based on core values, belief system in addition too learned behaviors along the way i.e. negative eating to seek comfort, over working to avoid family/partner disruptions.

To talk about identity is to talk about the condition character of being oneself Identity defines people and gives meaning to all aspect of their lives. It is shaped by life experiences past and present. "You determine who and what you will become". "Speak yourself into existence" aka tell yourself you can and you will, however you must take some action and responsibility for self. In short, you must know yourself, so you can set your life goals and self actualize. Positive self talk is vital to your emotional success in all areas of your life; you have the ability to do what ever it is you are willing to work at.

However, before you can begin the process of making changes to your identity with cognitive *(thinking)* or other techniques, you must first decide that exploring your identity is a worthwhile thing to do. FM is about making the mind, body and spirit connect to all aspects of your life, it about being willing to commit to your self for better long-term health, and maintain your desired weight goals, by taking back your personal power and control. Spirituality plays a major role in the human condition spirituality presents itself in many forms this varies from person to person, however, as human beings for the most part we seek the calming, loving source of energy, light within self or outside of self. This energy can express, manifest in any form you choose, this is a personal choice.

Meditation is a discipline in which one attempts to get beyond the conditioned, *thinking* mind into a deeper state of relaxation or awareness. It often involves turning attention to a single point of reference. Meditation is recognized as a component of almost all religions, and has been practiced for over 5,000 years. It is also practiced outside religious traditions. Different meditative disciplines encompass a wide range of spiritual and/or psychophysical practices which can emphasize different goals, from the achievement of a higher state of consciousness, to greater focus, creativity or self-awareness, or simply a more relaxed and peaceful frame of mind. The word *meditation* originally comes from the Indo-European root *med-*, meaning *to measure*. From the root *med-* are also derived the English words *mete, medicine, modest,* and *moderate.* It entered English as *meditation* through the Latin *meditatio*, which originally indicated every type of physical or intellectual exercise, then later evolved into the more specific meaning *contemplation* (Wikipedia online)

Meditation has been defined as: "self regulation of attention, in the service of self-inquiry, in the here and now." The various techniques of meditation can be classified according to their focus. Some focus on the field or background perception and experience, also called *mindfulness*; and others focus on a preselected specific object, and are called *concentrative* meditation. There are also techniques that shift between the field and the object. (Wikipedia online)

Breathing Meditation

1. Sit in a comfortable chair with your back straight and your feet flat on the floor. INHALE deeply and SLOWLY; as you EXHALE through your nose make a low humming sound if you choose.

2. In a quiet space free of any distractions, sit comfortably and close your eyes. Relax. This takes practice.

3. When your breath is EXHAUSTED, INHALE again and repeat; perform five cycles of this for a period of 2-3 minutes.

4. Initially start out with only 3-5 minutes, this is a gradual process due to the risk of hyperventilation because some people may breathe too deeply and fast. Practice makes better...practice, practice.

5. Breathe normally, but begin to focus your attention on the rhythm of your breath. Without trying to control or influence it in any way, become aware of air entering and leaving the body.

6. If your thoughts distract you, or you feel yourself becoming unfocused in any way, don't resist. Just allow your attention to come back to your breathing naturally.

7. Start small, 3-5 minutes, and gradually increase your time to practice relaxed breathing.

(Chopra Deepak. 2001. Overcoming Addictions; *the spiritual solution*)

LIGHT STRETCHING MEDITATION POSES/POSITIONS

ALWAYS STRECH YOUR BODY MUSCLES PRIOR TO ANY AND ALL PHYSICAL ACTIVITY
As you perform these exercises, remember to relax and assume the pose without force. Do not feel you have to execute each pose perfectly, Just strech your body to the point where you feel a gentle pressure;with practice and repetition you will become more flexible.

Vata balancing poses. Edited by Author please keep the shaded pictures

1. HEAD-TO-KNEE: This will take practice and patients on your part; you must always start with POSE 1 this is basic stretching along with focusing on your breathing. Sit on the floor with your legs stretched out in front of you. Bend your left knee and place the sole of your left foot flat against the inside of your right thigh. As you exhale, bend forward at the waist and reach to grasp your right foot with both hands. Don't strain, and allow yourself to bend your right knee slightly, if necessary. Try to avoid collapsing your chest or allowing your back to become overly round. Breathe normally, and hold this pose for a count of five. Return to a sitting posture and reverse the pose. Perform 3-5 cycles.

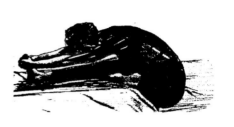

Vata balancing poses. Chopra Deepak. Overcoming Addictions; *the spiritual solution,* **2001.**

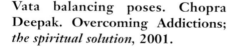

2. FORWARD BEND: Stand in a relaxed position with your arms comfortably at your sides. As you inhale, slowly raise your arms upward until they are starched above your head. Bend your head backwards until you feel a gentle stretch, and look upwards. Keeping your elbows straight and your hands extended bend forward at the waist and try to touch the floor in front of your toes. Stretch only as far as is comfortable, and don't feel you have to keep your knees locked. Remain bent at the waist for a count of five, and then return to a standing position as you inhale deeply repeats 3-5 times.

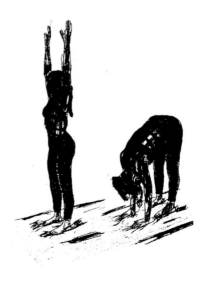

28

3. THUNDERBOLT POSE:

Kneel with your knees together and your weight resting back on your heels. Comfortably point your toes so that the soles of your feet face upward. Keep your back straight and your head up, and allow your hands to rest on your knees. Close your eyes and breathe deeply and evenly. Let your mind become clear. Maintain the pose for at least 30 seconds or for as long as is comfortable.

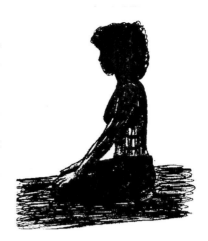

Vata balancing poses.

4. AWARENESS POSE:
Lie flat on your back with your palms open, facing upward beside your legs. Close your eyes and attempt to completely relax every area of your body. Breathe deeply, slowly rhythmically, and feel the tension disappearing from your muscles. True RELAXZATION is an art, and as you gain experience, confidence you'll feel yourself becoming more adept. The longer you practice focusing on your self without allowing outside interference i.e. phone, children, TV ect the purpose is total and complete focus on centering self to the point of being able to reduce pain, alleviate minor headaches.

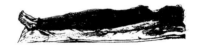

Vata balancing poses. Pictures edited by author please keep the shaded pictures

Let's Get Started

QUOTE FOR THE DAY

TODAY IS A NEW BEGINNING.

Let's get started taking back your power and control by taking action and practicing discipline. Once again, this is not about counting, weighing, and measuring, Let's start by planning your healthy low calorie meals. You know exactly how much you want to lose and/or maintain, so for the next 2-3 days, reflect on self, find two or more quotes that stand out, relate them to you, and begin to apply these statements as affirmations to yourself. Make yourself a schedule; include a stretching and meditation time and then begin to prepare your meats for your salads by baking chicken and/or turkey, and broiling salmon that you will eat at lunchtime daily. Due to the nutritional low calorie factor in salads, make it a large one with meat and cheese. The object is not to starve yourself, but to monitor how and what you eat, and to incorporate more physical activity into your daily routine.

    There are no food restrictions involved in food maintenance. This is about learning how to eat better, practicing self-discipline, learning to prepare healthier food, and to stop using/abusing food. Food maintenance is a way of living, Yes, you can have the nice slice of cake once a week, and make yourself one thick milkshake as well for a treat, using 2% milk. There is nothing you cannot eat; the only requirement is that you are willing to work for it. In addition, increase your water intake by 2-3 glasses of water per day to build up to 1 liter per day.

    Let's begin a new way of living healthier and thinking positively about your self. You can do anything once *YOU* make up your mind to do it. The daily quotes are meant to offer you encouragement and to assist you with a specific positive focus, or an area for change/improvement.

Physical Activities. Take the stairs at work as much as possible, go up and down your stairs at home, and start out doing three-five sit-ups once or twice a day. Start small and build up, but not too small; you know yourself and you know your heath. The object is not to overdo this and hurt yourself, it is to build you up because exercise requires consistency in order to be effective and burn calories. Use the eating and exercise logs to chart your progress and/or redirection. There is no pass or fail; if you fall off, getup. The hardest part is starting.

Using the Daily Schedule and Physical Activity/Positive Self-Talk. Example: Read the quote for the day and apply it to you or make your own. Physical Activities: I took the stairs all day at work today. This morning I did 5 minutes of mediation and some stretches, along with two situps and tonight I'll do 3-5 sit-ups.

Breakfast: 1 bowel of oatmeal with raisins, 1 Tbsp. of honey, store variety pack or regular oats with raisins, 1 C. of coffee, hard boil egg, O.J. or any juice. Don't forget to grab your liter of water for the day.

Lunch: Lg, salad with cheese, lettuce, broccoli, mushrooms, and chopped baked chicken, or turkey, or salmon, and a *lite* salad dressing. 1container of yogurt and 1 fruit.

Snack: Fresh fruit

Dinner: Modify your portions and make a vegetable salad and1 can of fruit cocktail or eat a large salad with baked meat, and 1 can of fruit cocktail. Snack on yogurt, increase your water intake, and have a low fat dessert.

Twice a week reward yourself. If Sunday dinner is the family meal, eat that nice slice of cake; you have been good all week, treat yourself. Also at any point during the week, please make yourself a thick milkshake with ice-cream and 2% Milk ONLY!

The Surgeon General's office estimates that obesity is responsible for some 300,000 deaths a year! It is imperative that you visit your doctor regularly, and have your cholesterol and blood pressure checked. High cholesterol and high blood pressure are *silent killers*. Pap smears and mammograms are musts in the battle against cancer. Always check with your physician regarding food and physical modifications in your regular routine. Take positive charge of your life.

Examples
Quote for Today:

DAILY SCHEDULE

Breakfast	
Lunch	
Snack	
Dinner	

PHYSICAL ACTIVITY/POSITIVE SELF-TALK

A.M.I did 5 minutes of mediation and stretches and completed 3 sit ups.	I took the stairs every other trip or I walked at lunch.	P.M. I did 3-5 sit-ups. I had a thick chocolate shake so I walked for 15 minutes, mediated and relaxed in the tub, played some relaxing music/gospel, instrumental, nature sounds.	
I will eat better today		I did better today. I feel good right now, in spite of the extra I ate. I walked for ten more minutes.	

This is an example of the types of things to record in your daily journal.

Progress NOT Perfection. One step at a time, one day at a time.

Quote for Today: I will begin today to practice self-care and love by eating better and walking 5-15 minutes today.

DAILY SCHEDULE DAY 1

Breakfast	
Lunch	
Snack	
Dinner	

PHYSICAL ACTIVITY/POSITIVE SELF-TALK

Remember, this is about *You*. *You* are the vital key person in this program. When you look for inspiration, care, and love you must first look within. No one has to tell you, you're alright today but you.

Progress NOT Perfection. One step at a time, one day at a time.

Quote for Today: Attitude determines attitude. (Unknown) please put the quote at the top of the page

DAILY SCHEDULE DAY 2

Breakfast	
Lunch	
Snack	
Dinner	

PHYSICAL ACTIVITY/POSITIVE SELF-TALK

Progress NOT Perfection. One step at a time, one day at a time.

Quote for Today: A man/woman sees in the world what he/she carries in his/her heart. (Opening scene of "Faust.")

DAILY SCHEDULE DAY 3

Breakfast	
Lunch	
Snack	
Dinner	

PHYSICAL ACTIVITY/POSITIVE SELF-TALK

Progress NOT Perfection. One step at a time, one day at a time.

Quote for Today: People don't care how much you know, until they know how much you care. (Unknown)

DAILY SCHEDULE DAY 4

Breakfast	
Lunch	
Snack	
Dinner	

PHYSICAL ACTIVITY/POSTIVE SELF-TALK

How do you feel? Don't look at the scale, that doesn't matter right now. We are concerned about developing better living and eating habits. Keep up the good work! We start out slow and build.

Progress NOT Perfection. One step at a time, one day at a time.

Quote for Today: No dreamer is ever too small; no dream is ever too big. (Unknown)

DAILY SCHEDULE DAY 5

Breakfast	
Lunch	
Snack	
Dinner	

PHYSICAL ACTIVITY/POSITIVE SELF-TALK

Progress NOT Perfection. One step at a time, one day at a time.

Quote for Today: To accomplish great things, we must not only dream; but act (Bill Blackman)

DAILY SCHEDULE DAY 6

Breakfast	
Lunch	
Snack	
Dinner	

PHYSICAL ACTIVITY/POSTIVE SELF-TALK

Progress NOT Perfection. One step at a time, one day at a time.

Quote for Today: Defeat is not defect unless accepted as a reality in your own mind. (Bruce Lee)

DAILY SCHEDULE DAY 7

Breakfast	
Lunch	
Snack	
Dinner	

PHYSICAL ACTIVITY/POSITIVE SELF-TALK

I love the queen's quote "a size Active"…she is amazing. Have you been able to convince a friend to get healthy? I always say, "I can show you better than I can tell you."

Progress NOT Perfection. One step at a time, one day at a time.

Quote for Today: Obstacles are those frightful things you see when you take your eyes off your goals. (Unknown)

DAILY SCHEDULE DAY 8

Breakfast	
Lunch	
Snack	
Dinner	

PHYSICAL ACTIVITY/POSTIVE SELF-TALK

Progress NOT Perfection. One step at a time, one day at a time.

Quote for Today: When you get to the end of your rope, tie a knot and hang on. (Franklin D Roosevelt)

DAILY SCHEDULE DAY 9

Breakfast	
Lunch	
Snack	
Dinner	

PHYSICAL ACTIVITY/POSITIVE SELF-TALK

How do you feel? Don't look at the scale, that doesn't matter right now. We are concerned about developing better living and eating habits. Keep up the good work! We start out slow and build.

Progress NOT Perfection. One step at a time, one day at a time.

Quote for Today: Our greatest glory is not in never failing, but in rising up every time we fail. (Ralph Waldo Emerson)

DAILY SCHEDULE DAY 10

Breakfast	
Lunch	
Snack	
Dinner	

PHYSICAL ACTIVITY/POSTIVE SELF-TALK

Progress NOT Perfection. One step at a time, one day at a time.

Quote for Today: Never, never, never give up. (Winston Churchill)

DAILY SCHEDULE DAY 11

Breakfast	
Lunch	
Snack	
Dinner	

PHYSICAL ACTIVITY/POSITIVE SELF-TALK

Progress NOT Perfection. One step at a time, one day at a time.

Quote for Today: And in the end, it's not the years in your life that count. It's the life in your years. (Abraham Lincoln)

DAILY SCHEDULE DAY 12

Breakfast	
Lunch	
Snack	
Dinner	

PHYSICAL ACTIVITY/POSTIVE SELF-TALK

Progress NOT Perfection. One step at a time, one day at a time.

Quote for Today: The secret of happiness is not in doing what one likes to do, but in liking what one has to do. (Unknown)

DAILY SCHEDULE DAY 13

Breakfast	
Lunch	
Snack	
Dinner	

PHYSICAL ACTIVITY/POSITIVE SELF-TALK

How do you feel? Don't look at the scale, that doesn't matter right now. We are concerned about developing better living and eating habits. Keep up the good work! We start out slow and build.

Progress NOT Perfection. One step at a time, one day at a time.

Quote for Today: The best and most beautiful things in this world cannot be seen or even heard, but must be felt with the heart (Helen Keller).

DAILY SCHEDULE DAY 14

Breakfast	
Lunch	
Snack	
Dinner	

PHYSICAL ACTIVITY/POSTIVE SELF-TALK

Are you feeling beautiful? You should be...you are a wonderful work in progress. Each day you develop you work and your program of better eating and living habits, while building yourself up. I applaud you in your efforts.

Progress NOT Perfection. One step at a time, one day at a time.

Quote for Today: People rarely succeed unless they have fun in what they are doing. (Dale Carnegie)

DAILY SCHEDULE DAY 15

Breakfast	
Lunch	
Snack	
Dinner	

PHYSICAL ACTIVITY/POSITIVE SELF-TALK

Progress NOT Perfection. One step at a time, one day at a time.

Quote for Today: Happiness is not a destination. It is a method of life. (Burton Hills)

DAILY SCHEDULE DAY 16

Breakfast	
Lunch	
Snack	
Dinner	

PHYSICAL ACTIVITY/POSTIVE SELF-TALK

Progress NOT Perfection. One step at a time, one day at a time.

Quote for Today: Dreams are renewable. No matter what our age or condition, there are still untapped possibilities within us and new beauty waiting to be born. (Dr. Dale Turner)

DAILY SCHEDULE DAY 17

Breakfast	
Lunch	
Snack	
Dinner	

PHYSICAL ACTIVITY/POSITIVE SELF-TALK

How do you feel? Don't look at the scale, that doesn't matter right now. We are concerned about developing better living and eating habits. Keep up the good work! We start out slow and build.

Progress NOT Perfection. One step at a time, one day at a time.

49

Quote for Today: Your thoughts are the architects of your destiny. (David O. McKay)

DAILY SCHEDULE DAY 18

Breakfast	
Lunch	
Snack	
Dinner	

PHYSICAL ACTIVITY/POSTIVE SELF-TALK

Progress NOT Perfection. One step at a time, one day at a time.

Quote for Today: When a man/woman finds no peace within self, it is useless to seek it elsewhere. (L.A. Rouchefolicauld)

DAILY SCHEDULE DAY 19

Breakfast	
Lunch	
Snack	
Dinner	

PHYSICAL ACTIVITY/POSITIVE SELF-TALK

How do you feel? Don't look at the scale, that doesn't matter right now. We are concerned about developing better living and eating habits. Keep up the good work! We start out slow and build.

.

Progress NOT Perfection. One step at a time, one day at a time.

Quote for Today: The most important of life's battles is the one we fight daily in the silent chambers of the soul. (David O. McKay)

DAILY SCHEDULE DAY 20

Breakfast	
Lunch	
Snack	
Dinner	

PHYSICAL ACTIVITY/POSTIVE SELF-TALK

Progress NOT Perfection. One step at a time, one day at a time.

Quote for Today: What lies behind us and what lies before us are tiny matters compared to what lies within us. (Unknown)

DAILY SCHEDULE DAY 21

Breakfast	
Lunch	
Snack	
Dinner	

PHYSICAL ACTIVITY/POSITIVE SELF TALK

Progress NOT Perfection. One step at a time, one day at a time.

Quote for Today: Are you fit company for the person you wish to become. (Unknown)

DAILY SCHEDULE DAY 22

Breakfast	
Lunch	
Snack	
Dinner	

PHYSICAL ACTIVITY/POSITIVE SELF TALK

How do you feel? Don't look at the scale, that doesn't matter right now. We are concerned about developing better living and eating habits. Keep up the good work! We start out slow and build.

Progress NOT Perfection. One step at a time, one day at a time.

Quote for Today: If you don't learn from your mistakes, there's no sense making them. (Unknown)

DAILY SCHEDULE DAY 23

Breakfast	
Lunch	
Snack	
Dinner	

PHYSICAL ACTIVITY/POSITIVE SELF TALK

Progress NOT Perfection. One step at a time, one day at a time.

Quote for Today: The biggest room in the world is room for improvement. (Unknown)

DAILY SCHEDULE DAY 24

Breakfast	
Lunch	
Snack	
Dinner	

PHYSICAL ACTIVITY/POSITIVE SELF TALK

Progress NOT Perfection. One step at a time, one day at a time.

Quote for Today: When we won't consider suggestions, we reject our own potential. (Bill Blackman)

DAILY SCHEDULE DAY 25

Breakfast	
Lunch	
Snack	
Dinner	

PHYSICAL ACTIVITY/POSITIVE SELF TALK

Progress NOT Perfection. One step at a time, one day at a time.

Quote for Today: Adversity is the diamond dust that heaven polishes its jewels with. (Leighton)

DAILY SCHEDULE DAY 26

Breakfast	
Lunch	
Snack	
Dinner	

PHYSICAL ACTIVITY/POSITIVE SELF TALK

Progress NOT Perfection. One step at a time, one day at a time.

Quote for Today: The storm also beats on the house that is built on the rock. (Unknown)

DAILY SCHEDULE DAY 27

Breakfast	
Lunch	
Snack	
Dinner	

PHYSICAL ACTIVITY/POSITIVE SELF TALK

Progress NOT Perfection. One step at a time, one day at a time.

Quote for Today: No one can make you feel inferior without your consent (Eleanor Roosevelt)

DAILY SCHEDULE DAY 28

Breakfast	
Lunch	
Snack	
Dinner	

PHYSICAL ACTIVITY/POSITIVE SELF TALK

Progress NOT Perfection. One step at a time, one day at a time.

Quote for Today: In order to be walked on, you have to be lying down. (Brian Weir)

DAILY SCHEDULE DAY 29

Breakfast	
Lunch	
Snack	
Dinner	

PHYSICAL ACTIVITY/POSITIVE SELF TALK

Progress NOT Perfection. One step at a time, one day at a time.

Quote for Today: I allow and welcome change. (Unknown)

DAILY SCHEDULE DAY 30

Breakfast	
Lunch	
Snack	
Dinner	

PHYSICAL ACTIVITY/POSITIVE SELF TALK

How do you feel? Don't look at the scale, that doesn't matter right now. We are concerned about developing better living and eating habits. Keep up the good work! We start out slow and build.

Progress NOT Perfection. One step at a time, one day at a time.

Quote for Today: I am willing to create new thoughts about my life and myself and how I choose to use food. (Unknown)

DAILY SCHEDULE DAY 31

Breakfast	
Lunch	
Snack	
Dinner	

PHYSICAL ACTIVITY/POSITIVE SELF TALK

Progress NOT Perfection. One step at a time, one day at a time.

Quote for Today: I am willing to go beyond my own limitations today. (Unknown)

DAILY SCHEDULE DAY 32

Breakfast	
Lunch	
Snack	
Dinner	

PHYSICAL ACTIVITY/POSITIVE SELF TALK

Progress NOT Perfection. One step at a time, one day at a time.

Quote for Today: My spiritual growth is proceeding day by day. (Unknown)

DAILY SCHEDULE DAY 33

Breakfast	
Lunch	
Snack	
Dinner	

PHYSICAL ACTIVITY/POSITIVE SELF TALK

Progress NOT Perfection. One step at a time, one day at a time.

Quote for Today: I am successful because I believed in me. (Unknown)

DAILY SCHEDULE DAY 34

Breakfast	
Lunch	
Snack	
Dinner	

PHYSICAL ACTIVITY/POSITIVE SELF TALK

Progress NOT Perfection. One step at a time, one day at a time.

Quote for Today: There is no right or wrong, I move beyond judgment. (Unknown)

DAILY SCHEDULE DAY 35

Breakfast	
Lunch	
Snack	
Dinner	

PHYSICAL ACTIVITY/POSITIVE SELF TALK

Progress NOT Perfection. One step at a time, one day at a time.

Quote for Today: I give myself permission to let go. (Unknown)

DAILY SCHEDULE DAY 36

Breakfast	
Lunch	
Snack	
Dinner	

PHYSICAL ACTIVITY/POSITIVE SELF TALK

Progress NOT Perfection. One step at a time, one day at a time.

Quote for Today: I accept peace. I have the power, strength, and knowledge today. (Unknown)

DAILY SCHEDULE DAY 37

Breakfast	
Lunch	
Snack	
Dinner	

PHYSICAL ACTIVITY/POSITIVE SELF TALK

Progress NOT Perfection. One step at a time, one day at a time.

Quote for Today: Love surrounds me and protects me and nourished me today. (Unknown)

DAILY SCHEDULE DAY 38

Breakfast	
Lunch	
Snack	
Dinner	

PHYSICAL ACTIVITY/POSITIVE SELF TALK

Progress NOT Perfection. One step at a time, one day at a time.

Quote for Today: I see myself with eyes of love. (Unknown)

DAILY SCHEDULE DAY 39

Breakfast	
Lunch	
Snack	
Dinner	

PHYSICAL ACTIVITY/POSITIVE SELF TALK

Progress NOT Perfection. One step at a time, one day at a time.

Quote for Today: I am free to be myself. (Unknown)

DAILY SCHEDULE DAY 40

Breakfast	
Lunch	
Snack	
Dinner	

PHYSICAL ACTIVITY/POSITIVE SELF TALK

Progress NOT Perfection. One step at a time, one day at a time.

Quote for Today: I love and embrace my uniqueiness today. (Unknown)

DAILY SCHEDULE DAY 41

Breakfast	
Lunch	
Snack	
Dinner	

PHYSICAL ACTIVITY/POSITIVE SELF TALK

How do you feel? Don't look at the scale, that doesn't matter right now. We are concerned about developing better living and eating habits. Keep up the good work! We start out slow and build.

Progress NOT Perfection. One step at a time, one day at a time.

Quote for Today: I am filled with positive energy and enthusiasm. (Unknown)

DAILY SCHEDULE DAY 42

Breakfast	
Lunch	
Snack	
Dinner	

PHYSICAL ACTIVITY/POSITIVE SELF TALK

Progress NOT Perfection. One step at a time, one day at a time.

Quote for Today: Good health is mine now. (Unknown)

DAILY SCHEDULE DAY 43

Breakfast	
Lunch	
Snack	
Dinner	

PHYSICAL ACTIVITY/POSITIVE SELF TALK

Progress NOT Perfection. One step at a time, one day at a time.

Quote for Today: My mind is at peace and all is well. (Unknown)

DAILY SCHEDULE DAY 44

Breakfast	
Lunch	
Snack	
Dinner	

PHYSICAL ACTIVITY/POSITIVE SELF TALK

Progress NOT Perfection. One step at a time, one day at a time.

Quote for Today: I give myself permission to be well. (Unknown)

DAILY SCHEDULE DAY 45

Breakfast	
Lunch	
Snack	
Dinner	

PHYSICAL ACTIVITY/POSITIVE SELF TALK

Progress NOT Perfection. One step at a time, one day at a time.

Quote for Today: I am gentle withmy body. I love myself today. (Unknown)

DAILY SCHEDULE DAY 46

Breakfast	
Lunch	
Snack	
Dinner	

PHYSICAL ACTIVITY/POSITIVE SELF TALK

Progress NOT Perfection. One step at a time, one day at a time.

Quote for Today: I will practice self-care and self-love. (Carmella)

DAILY SCHEDULE DAY 47

Breakfast	
Lunch	
Snack	
Dinner	

PHYSICAL ACTIVITY/POSITIVE SELF TALK

Progress NOT Perfection. One step at a time, one day at a time.

Quote for Today: I will develop better eating habits. (Carmella)

DAILY SCHEDULE DAY 48

Breakfast	
Lunch	
Snack	
Dinner	

PHYSICAL ACTIVITY/POSITIVE SELF TALK

Progress NOT Perfection. One step at a time, one day at a time.

Quote for Today: The perfection of my new way of living. (Unknown)

DAILY SCHEDULE DAY 49

Breakfast	
Lunch	
Snack	
Dinner	

PHYSICAL ACTIVITY/POSITIVE SELF TALK

Progress NOT Perfection. One step at a time, one day at a time.

Quote for Today: I relax and move with joy,ease, and comfort. (Unknown)

DAILY SCHEDULE DAY 50

Breakfast	
Lunch	
Snack	
Dinner	

PHYSICAL ACTIVITY/POSITIVE SELF TALK

How do you feel? Don't look at the scale, that doesn't matter right now. We are concerned about developing better living and eating habits. Keep up the good work! We start out slow and build.

Progress NOT Perfection. One step at a time, one day at a time.

Quote for Today: I am at home with the universe. (Unknown)

DAILY SCHEDULE DAY 51

Breakfast	
Lunch	
Snack	
Dinner	

PHYSICAL ACTIVITY/POSITIVE SELF TALK

Progress NOT Perfection. One step at a time, one day at a time.

Quote for Today: I must work on changing my way of living. (Unknown)

DAILY SCHEDULE DAY 52

Breakfast	
Lunch	
Snack	
Dinner	

PHYSICAL ACTIVITY/POSITIVE SELF TALK

Progress NOT Perfection. One step at a time, one day at a time.

Quote for Today: I must continue to work on my better eating/living habits. (Carmella)

DAILY SCHEDULE DAY 53

Breakfast	
Lunch	
Snack	
Dinner	

PHYSICAL ACTIVITY/POSITIVE SELF TALK

Progress NOT Perfection. One step at a time, one day at a time.

Quote for Today: I now go beyond my old fears and limitations. (Unknown)

DAILY SCHEDULE DAY 54

Breakfast	
Lunch	
Snack	
Dinner	

PHYSICAL ACTIVITY/POSITIVE SELF TALK

Progress NOT Perfection. One step at a time, one day at a time.

Quote for Today: My inner vision is clear. (Unknown)

DAILY SCHEDULE DAY 55

Breakfast	
Lunch	
Snack	
Dinner	

PHYSICAL ACTIVITY/POSITIVE SELF TALK

Progress NOT Perfection. One step at a time, one day at a time.

Quote for Today: I am powerful and capable. I love and appreciate all of myself. (Unknown)

DAILY SCHEDULE DAY 56

Breakfast	
Lunch	
Snack	
Dinner	

PHYSICAL ACTIVITY/POSITIVE SELF TALK

Progress NOT Perfection. One step at a time, one day at a time.

Quote for Today: It's easy to live for others. I call on you to live for yourself. (Ralph W. Emerson)

DAILY SCHEDULE DAY 57

Breakfast	
Lunch	
Snack	
Dinner	

PHYSICAL ACTIVITY/POSITIVE SELF TALK

Progress NOT Perfection. One step at a time, one day at a time.

Quote for Today: Prayer begins where our powers ends. (Rabbi Abraham Heschel)

DAILY SCHEDULE DAY 58

Breakfast	
Lunch	
Snack	
Dinner	

PHYSICAL ACTIVITY/POSITIVE SELF TALK

Progress NOT Perfection. One step at a time, one day at a time.

Quote for Today: Wherever you go, there you are. (Earnie Larsen)

DAILY SCHEDULE DAY 59

Breakfast	
Lunch	
Snack	
Dinner	

PHYSICAL ACTIVITY/POSITIVE SELF TALK

Progress NOT Perfection. One step at a time, one day at a time.

Quote for Today: No one has time; we have to make time. (James Rhoen)

DAILY SCHEDULE DAY 60

Breakfast	
Lunch	
Snack	
Dinner	

PHYSICAL ACTIVITY/POSITIVE SELF TALK

Progress NOT Perfection. One step at a time, one day at a time.

Quote for Today: The best is yet to be. (Robert Browning)

DAILY SCHEDULE DAY 61

Breakfast	
Lunch	
Snack	
Dinner	

PHYSICAL ACTIVITY/POSITIVE SELF TALK

Progress NOT Perfection. One step at a time, one day at a time.

Quote for Today: Be yourself. (The Desiderata)

DAILY SCHEDULE DAY 62

Breakfast	
Lunch	
Snack	
Dinner	

PHYSICAL ACTIVITY/POSITIVE SELF TALK

Progress NOT Perfection. One step at a time, one day at a time.

Quote for Today: Anger is not evil. It is simply power waiting to be directed. (S. Dale Smith)

DAILY SCHEDULE DAY 63

Breakfast	
Lunch	
Snack	
Dinner	

PHYSICAL ACTIVITY/POSITIVE SELF TALK

How do you feel? Don't look at the scale, that doesn't matter right now. We are concerned about developing better living and eating habits. Keep up the good work! We start out slow and build.

Progress NOT Perfection. One step at a time, one day at a time.

Quote for Today: Most of what we want to be, we already are. (Kevin K.)

DAILY SCHEDULE DAY 64

Breakfast	
Lunch	
Snack	
Dinner	

PHYSICAL ACTIVITY/POSITIVE SELF TALK

Progress NOT Perfection. One step at a time, one day at a time.

Quote for Today: Character consists of what you do on the third or fourth tries. (James Michener)

DAILY SCHEDULE DAY 65

Breakfast	
Lunch	
Snack	
Dinner	

PHYSICAL ACTIVITY/POSITIVE SELF TALK

Progress NOT Perfection. One step at a time, one day at a time.

Quote for Today: You must motivate yourself EVERYDAY. (Matthew Stasior)

DAILY SCHEDULE DAY 66

Breakfast	
Lunch	
Snack	
Dinner	

PHYSICAL ACTIVITY/POSITIVE SELF TALK

Progress NOT Perfection. One step at a time, one day at a time.

Quote for Today: Change your thoughts and you change your world. (Norman Vincent Peale)

DAILY SCHEDULE DAY 67

Breakfast	
Lunch	
Snack	
Dinner	

PHYSICAL ACTIVITY/POSITIVE SELF TALK

Progress NOT Perfection. One step at a time, one day at a time.

Quote for Today: I am responsible for my experiences. (Unknown)

DAILY SCHEDULE DAY 68

Breakfast	
Lunch	
Snack	
Dinner	

PHYSICAL ACTIVITY/POSITIVE SELF TALK

Progress NOT Perfection. One step at a time, one day at a time.

Quote for Today: The best motivation always comes from within. (Michael Johnson)

DAILY SCHEDULE DAY 69

Breakfast	
Lunch	
Snack	
Dinner	

PHYSICAL ACTIVITY/POSITIVE SELF TALK

Progress NOT Perfection. One step at a time, one day at a time.

Quote for Today: They always say time changes things, but you actually have to change them yourself. (Andy Warhol)

DAILY SCHEDULE DAY 70

Breakfast	
Lunch	
Snack	
Dinner	

PHYSICAL ACTIVITY/POSITIVE SELF TALK

Progress NOT Perfection. One step at a time, one day at a time.

Quote for Today: These are only thoughts and thoughts can be changed. (Unknown)

DAILY SCHEDULE DAY 71

Breakfast	
Lunch	
Snack	
Dinner	

PHYSICAL ACTIVITY/POSITIVE SELF TALK

Progress NOT Perfection. One step at a time, one day at a time.

Quote for Today: Only I can change my life. No one can do it for me. (Carol Burnett)

DAILY SCHEDULE DAY 72

Breakfast	
Lunch	
Snack	
Dinner	

PHYSICAL ACTIVITY/POSITIVE SELF TALK

Progress NOT Perfection. One step at a time, one day at a time.

Quote for Today: I deserve good heath. (Unknown)

DAILY SCHEDULE DAY 73

Breakfast	
Lunch	
Snack	
Dinner	

PHYSICAL ACTIVITY/POSITIVE SELF TALK

Progress NOT Perfection. One step at a time, one day at a time.

Quote for Today: The point of power is now. (Unknown)

DAILY SCHEDULE DAY 74

Breakfast	
Lunch	
Snack	
Dinner	

PHYSICAL ACTIVITY/POSITIVE SELF TALK

Progress NOT Perfection. One step at a time, one day at a time.

Quote for Today: We all have big changes in our lives that are more or less a second chance. (Harrison Ford)

DAILY SCHEDULE DAY 75

Breakfast	
Lunch	
Snack	
Dinner	

PHYSICAL ACTIVITY/POSITIVE SELF TALK

Progress NOT Perfection. One step at a time, one day at a time.

Quote for Today: I listen to my body's needs. (Unknown)

DAILY SCHEDULE DAY 76

Breakfast	
Lunch	
Snack	
Dinner	

PHYSICAL ACTIVITY/POSITIVE SELF TALK

Progress NOT Perfection. One step at a time, one day at a time.

Quote for Today: Whoever said anybody has a right to give up? (Marian Wright Edelman)

DAILY SCHEDULE DAY 77

Breakfast	
Lunch	
Snack	
Dinner	

PHYSICAL ACTIVITY/POSITIVE SELF TALK

Progress NOT Perfection. One step at a time, one day at a time.

Quote for Today: Life is a great big canvas, and you should throw all the paint you can on it. (Danny Kaye)

DAILY SCHEDULE DAY 78

Breakfast	
Lunch	
Snack	
Dinner	

PHYSICAL ACTIVITY/POSITIVE SELF TALK

Progress NOT Perfection. One step at a time, one day at a time.

Quote for Today: Action is the antidote to despair. (Joan Baez)

DAILY SCHEDULE DAY 79

Breakfast	
Lunch	
Snack	
Dinner	

PHYSICAL ACTIVITY/POSITIVE SELF TALK

Progress NOT Perfection. One step at a time, one day at a time.

Quote for Today: Failure is only the opportunity to begin again, this time more wisely. (Anonymous)

DAILY SCHEDULE DAY 80

Breakfast	
Lunch	
Snack	
Dinner	

PHYSICAL ACTIVITY/POSITIVE SELF TALK

Progress NOT Perfection. One step at a time, one day at a time.

Quote for Today: Actions speak louder than words. (English Proverb)

DAILY SCHEDULE DAY 81

Breakfast	
Lunch	
Snack	
Dinner	

PHYSICAL ACTIVITY/POSITIVE SELF TALK

Progress NOT Perfection. One step at a time, one day at a time.

Quote for Today: Not being able to do everything is no excuse for not doing everything you can. (Ashleigh Brilliant)

DAILY SCHEDULE DAY 82

Breakfast	
Lunch	
Snack	
Dinner	

PHYSICAL ACTIVITY/POSITIVE SELF TALK

Progress NOT Perfection. One step at a time, one day at a time.

Quote for Today: The journey of a thousand miles must begin with a single step. (Lao Tzu)

DAILY SCHEDULE DAY 83

Breakfast	
Lunch	
Snack	
Dinner	

PHYSICAL ACTIVITY/POSITIVE SELF TALK

How do you feel? Don't look at the scale, that doesn't matter right now. We are concerned about developing better living and eating habits. Keep up the good work! We start out slow and build.

Progress NOT Perfection. One step at a time, one day at a time.

115

Quote for Today: Great changes may not happen right away, but with effort even the difficult may become easy. (Bill Blackman)

DAILY SCHEDULE DAY 84

Breakfast	
Lunch	
Snack	
Dinner	

PHYSICAL ACTIVITY/POSITIVE SELF TALK

Progress NOT Perfection. One step at a time, one day at a time.

Quote for Today: The beginning is the half of every action. (Greek Proverb)

DAILY SCHEDULE DAY 85

Breakfast	
Lunch	
Snack	
Dinner	

PHYSICAL ACTIVITY/POSITIVE SELF TALK

Progress NOT Perfection. One step at a time, one day at a time.

Quote for Today: Unite to move forward. (American Proverb)

DAILY SCHEDULE DAY 86

Breakfast	
Lunch	
Snack	
Dinner	

PHYSICAL ACTIVITY/POSITIVE SELF TALK

At this point have you asked family or friends to get active with you or have you started a lunch time walk with co-workers.

Progress NOT Perfection. One step at a time, one day at a time.

Quote for Today: Progress is the activity of today and the assurance of tomorrow. (Ralph Waldo Emerson)

DAILY SCHEDULE DAY 87

Breakfast	
Lunch	
Snack	
Dinner	

PHYSICAL ACTIVITY/POSITIVE SELF TALK

Progress NOT Perfection. One step at a time, one day at a time.

Quote for Today: If there is no struggle, there is no progress. (Frederick Douglass)

DAILY SCHEDULE DAY 88

Breakfast	
Lunch	
Snack	
Dinner	

PHYSICAL ACTIVITY/POSITIVE SELF TALK

Progress NOT Perfection. One step at a time, one day at a time.

Quote for Today: All progress occurs because people dare to be different. (Harry Milner)

DAILY SCHEDULE DAY 89

Breakfast	
Lunch	
Snack	
Dinner	

PHYSICAL ACTIVITY/POSITIVE SELF TALK

How do you feel? Are you ready to look at the scale just too see how well your doing.

Progress NOT Perfection. One step at a time, one day at a time.

Quote for Today: True progress quietly and persistently moves along without notice. (St. Francis of Assisi)

DAILY SCHEDULE DAY 90

Breakfast	
Lunch	
Snack	
Dinner	

PHYSICAL ACTIVITY/POSITIVE SELF TALK

Progress NOT Perfection. One step at a time, one day at a time.

Quote for Today: To succeed, you need to take that gut feeling in what you believe and act on it with all of your heart. (Christy Borgeld)

DAILY SCHEDULE DAY 91

Breakfast	
Lunch	
Snack	
Dinner	

PHYSICAL ACTIVITY/POSITIVE SELF TALK

Progress NOT Perfection. One step at a time, one day at a time.

Quote for Today: To freely bloom - that is my definition of success. (Gerry Spence)

DAILY SCHEDULE DAY 92

Breakfast	
Lunch	
Snack	
Dinner	

PHYSICAL ACTIVITY/POSITIVE SELF TALK

Progress NOT Perfection. One step at a time, one day at a time.

Quote for Today: Discipline is the bridge between goals and accomplishment. (Jim Rohn)

DAILY SCHEDULE DAY 93

Breakfast	
Lunch	
Snack	
Dinner	

PHYSICAL ACTIVITY/POSITIVE SELF TALK

Progress NOT Perfection. One step at a time, one day at a time.

Quote for Today: We mustn't let our passions destroy our dreams. (Anonymous)

DAILY SCHEDULE DAY 94

Breakfast	
Lunch	
Snack	
Dinner	

PHYSICAL ACTIVITY/POSITIVE SELF TALK

Progress NOT Perfection. One step at a time, one day at a time.

Quote for Today: It is easier to suppress the first desire than to satisfy all that follow. (Anonymous)

DAILY SCHEDULE DAY 95

Breakfast	
Lunch	
Snack	
Dinner	

PHYSICAL ACTIVITY/POSITIVE SELF TALK

Progress NOT Perfection. One step at a time, one day at a time.

Quote for Today: There is no pleasure in life equal to that of the conquest of a vicious habit. (Anonymous)

DAILY SCHEDULE DAY 96

Breakfast	
Lunch	
Snack	
Dinner	

PHYSICAL ACTIVITY/POSITIVE SELF TALK

Progress NOT Perfection. One step at a time, one day at a time.

Quote for Today: There is no luck except where there is discipline. (Irish Proverb)

DAILY SCHEDULE DAY 97

Breakfast	
Lunch	
Snack	
Dinner	

PHYSICAL ACTIVITY/POSITIVE SELF TALK

Progress NOT Perfection. One step at a time, one day at a time.

Quote for Today: He who conquers himself has won a greater victory than he who conquers a city. (Proverbs)

DAILY SCHEDULE DAY 98

Breakfast	
Lunch	
Snack	
Dinner	

PHYSICAL ACTIVITY/POSITIVE SELF TALK

Progress NOT Perfection. One step at a time, one day at a time.

Quote for Today: You can, you have, and you will continue to be the wonderful healthier you. (Carmella)

DAILY SCHEDULE DAY 99

Breakfast	
Lunch	
Snack	
Dinner	

PHYSICAL ACTIVITY/POSITIVE SELF TALK

Progress NOT Perfection. One step at a time, one day at a time.

Quote for Today: Real glory springs from the silent conquest of ourselves. (Anonymous)

DAILY SCHEDULE DAY 100

Breakfast	
Lunch	
Snack	
Dinner	

PHYSICAL ACTIVITY/POSITIVE SELF TALK

Progress NOT Perfection. One step at a time, one day at a time.

SO! How do you feel now that you have completed your first 100 days of better eating and living habits, while incorperating situps in your daily schedule? Are you surprised? I'm not; you started out small and have gradually built yourself up. Look back at your progress; I know you feel good about you, and I know you look good too. So, tell me, are you going to throw out the scale now that you are practicing better eating habits and telling yourself, *I can eat anything I choose as long as I'm willing to work for it?* If you are up to 30 sit-ups twice a day, and you are walking a mile in a day or two, you are golden. The walking doesn't have to be in the park. The workplace is just as good; take the stairs as much as possible and, if you made time in your schedule to walk, good girl.

Congratulations! I have stayed with you long enough; practice what you learned here, take the information to heart, and continue to apply it to your life. And by all means, please continue to use this guideline for the *next* 100 days.

BREATHE EASY
(KAMEISHA)

breathe easy ""'"
you sofly whisper, you are wonderful"" and with each step you take
the world creeks with fear, never knowing what to expect
you think you might fall, but love always hear the unspoken
words of the heart and you are safe with me.

no more blank pages, its your chance take control
you assumed wrong, regret is long gone so
leave the stairs, you didn't get to climb, Be bold
and borrow my strength; you too will endure the storm
that seems to have end, but in me you always have a friend

you're learning while your giving yourself a chance to grow
dream while our awake, but open your heart to all that life
Will bring, scream if you must, but be happy with what you see
don't watch for take place, live in the moments that makes you smile
love will always hear the unspoken words.

the world is no longer there ,,,, and tears like rain
Will pour, you will never be the same, not any more
you've given yourself the chance to change
and finally you are able to live
because many people care and are starting to share
love hears the words unspoken

now you ask, could this be has love really found me
no more doubts or sothered gray clouds
my love that you've taken, is sure and not mistaken
and is because you believed in you, write the end of
your own love and faith, love always hear the words unspoken.

(Kameisha)

Thank you for purchasing this book; it is my goal to inspire and empower those that feel powerless for whatever reason. My focus and reason for this book is a sister/friend died in 2005 at the age of 44 due to compulsive overeating; she literally ate herself to death, due to long-term negative eating habits and negative family situations. My sister abuses food as well, and she has medical complications as a result of her long-term overeating behaviors.

In conjunction with my past substance dependence, I was unable to intervene and assist because I was emotionally and mentally impaired. I missed the opportunity to help my own; but maybe I can help others by communicating with you all through this book. It's been a long road home, but I'm home now, and my heart is into promoting a healthy you from the inside out.

Love and healing start and grow from within; I ask you all to seek out some form of spirituality, in order to fill the void in your life and reduce the risk of relapsing on food by continuing the unhealthy eating behavior in crisis situations and/or family pressure. If you find at some point during the reading of the materials in this book that you need additional services, I encourage you to seek that out and have regular physical checkups. Self-care is vital to all human kind, and my personal opinion is simply if I cannot take good care of me, how then can I take care of you when I'm sick.

About the Author

I'm 44 year-old African American woman, I have one daughter she is 13 she is my heart beat, my piece of heaven on earth. I have a degree in Counseling and I'm an GPN, I'm a grateful recovering substance user, and I understand the basic dynamic of using substances, i.e. drugs, food, alcohol, and sex as a means of filling that internal void, and through my healing process, I have watched others substitute one thing for the another until the pain became so great that internal change had to be made. Personal health and growth starts from within. I thank GOD for blessing me and my family.

Carmella & daughter Charnell

Inspirational Quotes

1. Never giving up and pushing forward will unlock all the potential we are capable of. (Christy Borgeld)

2. Adventure is worthwhile. (Amelia Earhart)

3. Now is the time. Needs are great, but your possibilities are greater. (Bill Blackman)

4. Courage faces fear and thereby masters it. (Martin Luther King, Jr.)

5. Challenges are what make life interesting; overcoming them is what makes life meaningful. (Joshua J. Marine)

6. To go against the dominant thinking of your friends, of most of the people you see every day, is perhaps the most difficult act of heroism you can perform. (Theodore H. White)

7. Difficulties are meant to rouse, not discourage. The human spirit is to grow strong by conflict. (William Ellery Channing)

8. A hero gets scared, but still goes on. (Anonymous)

9. Accept challenges, so that you may feel the exhilaration of victory. (George S. Patton)

10. You gain strength, courage, and confidence by every experience in which you really stop to look fear in the face. You must do the thing which you think you cannot do. (Eleanor Roosevelt)

11. Health and intellect are the two blessings of life. (Menander)

12. Who indeed can harm you if you are committed deeply to doing what is right? (I Peter)

13. Health and cheerfulness naturally beget each other. (Joseph Addison).

14. People are like stained-glass windows. They sparkle and shine when the sun is out, but when the darkness sets in their true beauty is revealed only if there is a light from within. (Elisabeth Kubler-Ross)

15. Every human being is the author of your own health

16. Everything has beauty, but not everyone sees it. (Confucius)

17. Nothing is more fatal to health than an over care of it. (Benjamin Franklin)

18. Happiness is a state of activity. (Aristotle)

19. Life expectancy would grow by leaps and bounds if green vegetables smelled as good as bacon. (Doug Larson)

20. People often say that 'beauty is in the eye of the beholder,' and I say that the most liberating thing about beauty is realizing that you are the beholder. This empowers us to find beauty in places where others have not dared to look, including inside ourselves. (Salma Hayek)

21. To wish to be well is part of becoming well. (Seneca)

22. A good laugh and a long sleep are the best cures in the doctor's book. (Irish Proverb)

23. What worth has beauty if it is not seen? (Italian Proverb)

24. The greatest wealth is health. (Virgil)

25. Beauty is not so much what you see as what you dream. (Walloon Proverb)

26. One must eat to live and not live to eat. (Moliere)

27. Attitude determines attitude. (Unknown)

28. Life without a purpose is a languid, drifting thing; every day we ought to review our purpose, saying to ourselves, 'This day let me make a sound beginning.' (Thomas Kempis)

29. A man/woman sees in the world what he/she carries in his/her heart (Opening scene of "Faust")

30. People don't care how much you know, until they know how much you care. (Unknown)

31. No dreamer is ever too small; no dream is ever too big. (Unknown)

32. To accomplish great things, we must not only dream; but act. (Bill Blackman)

33. Defeat is not defect unless accepted as a reality in your own mind.(Bruce Lee)

34. Obstacles are those frightful things you see when you take your eyes off your goals. (Unknown)

35. When you get to the end of your rope, tie a knot and hang on. (Franklin D. Roosevelt)

36. Our greatest glory is in never failing, but in rising up every time we fail. (Ralph Waldo Emerson)

37. Never, never, never give up. (Winston Churchill)

38. The biggest room in the world is room for improvement. (Unknown)

39. And, in the end it's not the years in your life that count. It's the life in your years. (Abraham Lincoln)

40. The secret of happiness is not in doing what one likes to do, but in liking what one has to do. (Unknown)

41. The best and most beautiful things in this world cannot be seen or even heard, but must be felt with the heart (Helen Keller)

42. I am successful because I believed in me. (Unknown)

43. People rarely succeed unless they have fun in what they are doing. (Dale Carnegie)

44. Happiness is not a destination. It is a method of life. (Burton Hills)

45. Dreams are renewable. No matter what our age or condition, there are still untapped possibilities within us and new beauty waiting to be born. (Dr. Dale Turner)

46. Your thoughts are the architects of your destiny. (David O. McKay)

47. When a man/woman finds no peace within self, it is useless to seek it elsewhere. (L.A. Rouchefolicauld)

48. The most important of life's battles is the one we fight daily in the silent chambers of the soul. (David O. McKay)

49. What lies behind us and what lies before us are tiny matters compared to what lies within us. (Unknown)

50. Are you fit company for the person you wish to become. (Unknown)

51. If you don't learn from your mistakes, there's no sense making them. (Unknown)

52. When we won't consider suggestions, we reject our own potential. (Bill Blackman)

53. Adversity is the diamond dust that heaven polishes its jewels with. (Leighton)

54. The storm also beats on the house that is built on the rock. (Unknown)

55. No one can make you feel inferior without your consent (Eleanor Roosevelt)

56. In order to be walked on, you have to be lying down. (Brian Weir)

57. I allow and welcome change. (Unknown)

58. I am willing to create new thoughts about my life and myself and how I choose to use food. (Unknown)

59. I am willing to go beyond my own limitations today. (Unknown)

60. My spiritual growth is proceeding day by day. (Unknown)

140

61. There is no right or wrong, I move beyond judgment. (Unknown)

62. I give myself permission to let go. (Unknown)

63. I accept peace. I have the power, strength, and knowledge today (Unknown)

64. Love surrounds me and protects me and nourished me today. (Unknown)

65. I love and embrace my uniqueiness today. (Unknown)

66. The best motivation always comes from within. (Michael Johnson)

67. I am filled with positive energy, and enthusiasm. (Unknown)

68. Good health is mine now. (Unknown)

69. My mind is at peace and all is well. (Unknown)

70. The perfection of my new way of living. (Unknown)

71. I relax and move with joy, ease, and comfort. (Unknown)

72. My inner vision is clear. (Unknown)

73. It's easy to live for others. I call on you to live for yourself. (Ralph W. Emerson)

74. Prayer begins where our power ends. (Rabbi Abraham Heschel)

75. Wherever you go, there you are. (Earnie Larsen)

76. No one has time; we have to make time. (James Rhoen)

77. The best is yet to be. (Robert Browning)

78. Be yourself. (The Desiderata)

79. Anger is not evil. It is simply power waiting to be directed (S. Dale Smith)

80. Most of what we want to be, we already are. (Kevin K.)

81. Character consists of what you do on the third or fourth tries. (James Michener)

141

82. You must motivate yourself everyday. (Matthew Stasior)

83. Action is the antidote to despair. (Joan Baez)

84. Change your thoughts and you change your world. (Norman Vincent Peale)

85. They always say time changes things, but you actually have to change them yourself. (Andy Warhol)

86. Only I can change my life. No one can do it for me. (Carol Burnett)

87. The point of power is now. (Unknown)

88. We all have big changes in our lives that are more or less a second chance. (Harrison Ford)

89. Whoever said anybody has a right to give up? (Marian Wright Edelman)

90. Actions speak louder than words. (English Proverb)

91. Life is a great big canvas, and you should throw all the paint you can on it. (Danny Kaye)

92. Action is the antidote to despair. (Joan Baez)

93. Failure is only the opportunity to begin again, this time more wisely. (Anonymous)

94. Not being able to do everything is no excuse for not doing everything you can. (Ashleigh Brilliant)

95. The journey of a thousand miles must begin with a single step. (Lao Tzu)

96. Great changes may not happen right away, but with effort even the difficult may become easy. (Bill Blackman)

97. The beginning is the half of every action. (Greek Proverb)

98. Unite to move forward. (American Proverb)

99. Progress is the activity of today and the assurance of tomorrow. (Ralph Waldo Emerson)

100. If there is no struggle, there is no progress. (Frederick Douglass)

101. All progress occurs because people dare to be different. (Harry Milner)

102. True progress quietly and persistently moves along without notice (St. Francis of Assisi)

103. To succeed, you need to take that gut feeling in what you believe and act on it with all of your heart. (Christy Borgeld)

104. To freely bloom - that is my definition of success. (Gerry Spence)

105. Discipline is the bridge between goals and accomplishment. (Jim Rohn)

106. We mustn't let our passions destroy our dreams. (Anonymous)

107. It is easier to suppress the first desire than to satisfy all that follow. (Anonymous)

108. There is no pleasure in life equal to that of the conquest of a vicious habit. (Anonymous)

109. There is no luck except where there is discipline. (Irish Proverb)

110. He who conquers himself has won a greater victory than he who conquers a city. (Proverbs)

111. Real glory springs from the silent conquest of ourselves. (Anonymous)

Sources

1. Vata balancing poses, and The Ayurveda Mind Body Questionnaire Chopra Deepak. Overcoming Addictions; *the spiritual solution* New York Harmony Books, 2001.
2. Poems (Original) Reaching Within Author Carmella Irick
3. Poems (Original) Breath Easy Kameisha
   All other online sources listed below:
4. All Quotations are cited from online source www.heartsandmind.org
5. Nutrition
6. Ayurveda Holistic Health Information cited from (On-line source wikipedia.org)
7. (Original source) Ayurveda Holistic Health Information Wujastyk, D. (2003). *The Roots of Ayurveda: Selections from Sanskrit Medical Writings.* Penguin Classics:
8. Chopra, A.S. (2003) in "Ayurveda", *Medicine Across Cultures*, edited by Selin, Helaine & Shapiro, H. 75-83. Kluwer Academic Publishers. United States of America:
9. Dwivedi, Girish & Dwivedi, Shridhar (2007). *History of Medicine: Sushruta – the Clinician – Teacher par Excellence*. National Informatics Centre (Government of India).
10. Clip Art, AOL
11. Wrongdiagnosis. com Statistics about Overweight & Associated Conditions for Overweight
12. Women's Heart Foundation (WHF) women's heart health information
13. Overeater Questionnaire and general infoirmationwww.oa.org
14. Overweight and Obesity Statistics: American Heart Association, americanheart.org./ Original *Source: MMWR Surveill Summ. 2006; 55:1-108.).*